SJOGREN'S SYNDROME:

the

SNEAKY

"ARTHRITIS"

by

SUE DAUPHIN

Copyright © Sue Dauphin 1987

All rights reserved. No part of this book may be reproduced or transmitted in any form or by any means, electronic or mechanical, including photocopying, recording or by any information storage and retrieval system without written permission of the author, except for the inclusion of brief quotations in critical articles and reviews.

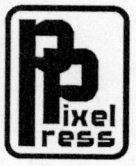

P.O.Box 3151
Tequesta, Florida, 33469-0151

Printed in the United States of America

Library of Congress Catalog Card Number: 88-90652

ISBN 0-9620354-0-8

TABLE OF CONTENTS

Illustrations

Preface

Foreword

Ch.	I	Introduction/Definition	1
	2	Symptoms	15
	3	Immunology	43
	4	History	55
	5	Diagnosis/Testing	61
	6	Treatment	73
	7	Research	103
	8	Prognosis/Support Resources	111
	9	Conclusion	123

Glossary 129

Bibliography 139

Index 149

ACKNOWLEDGEMENTS

There are many people without whose help this book could not have been written. Chief among them are the doctors and research scientists who gave of their valuable time to offer advice, encouragement, and most importantly, information. They include Dr. Elaine Alexander, Dr. Frank Arnett, Dr. Anna Ballestra, Dr. Troy Daniels, Dr. John Egerton, Dr. Robert J. Kassan, Dr. Seymour Katz, Dr. H. M. Moutsopoulos, Dr. Susumi Sugai, Dr. Norman Talal, Dr. Carmac Taylor, Dr. John Whelton and the many others whose writings informed my research.

Special thanks go to Lottie Bluesteen, Sara Brown, Sister Eleanor Dickman, Sara Endress, Bridget Fuchs, Elaine Harris, Doris Heath, Lucille Johnson, Bernice Kapalin, Aileen Lull, Dan Morales, Mrs. M. Rapps, Doris Reprogel, Betty Rosen, Helen Ruhl, Jane Tarail, Rose Thomas, and Betty Willert, patient/members of Sjogren's Syndrome Foundation Chapters who shared their experiences with me. Also invaluable were the publications of The Sjogren's Syndrome Foundation and the Arthritis Foundation. Technical editor Arthur R. Harris, was particularly indispensable.

None of these would have been enough without the loving support and many contributions of my husband, Vern.

It may be noted that there is a preponderance of women among the patients acknowledged here. This holds true throughout this book, mainly because it is also true among the general population of Sjogren's syndrome patients. To ward off any indignation on this point, I will use "he" or "she" interchangeably in my text in referring to both patients and doctors.

LIST OF ILLUSTRATIONS

Figure	1	Cheeks Like a Chipmunk	6
	2	Tear Ducts and Glands	16
	3	Eyeball showing 3 Layer Tear Film	17
	4	Salivary Glands	22
	5	Lymph Nodes for Self-Examination	33
	6	Figure Showing Complaints	41
	7	Figure Unmarked for Reader	42
	8	Factors in Autoimmunity	48
	9	Sjogren's Syndrome Diagnostic Criteria Compared	66
	10	Schirmer Test	67
	11	Medications That May Cause Dry Eyes or Mouth	69
	12	Artificial Tear Ingredients	74
	13	Reservoir Glasses	76
	14	Too Many Milkshakes!	79
	15	Lemon Peel Stimulating Saliva	81
	16	NSAIDs with Side Effects	83
	17	Joint with Synovial Capsule	88
	18	Walkin' and Talkin'	91
	19	Moisturizers	94
	20	Quack Selling "Joint Oil"	100
	21	Paracelsus Planting "Mummified" Magnet Seeds	102
	22	The Rare SS Bird	113

PREFACE

<u>Someone you know may be hurting and not know why.</u>
He or she belongs to a "chapter" of the reluctant fraternity of an estimated 36 million Americans who suffer from arthritis. Worldwide, it's estimated that many more than 3% of the population have some type of auto-immune disease. **More than 4 million** of those are thought to have a disorder known as Sjogren's syndrome. But most have never been diagnosed. Far too many doctors don't recognize it when they see it.

Some patients go 20 years or more before getting a name to hang on to their affliction. Often they are labeled hypochondriacs. Their mouths are dry. There's 'something in their eyes'. Their joints hurt. They have that 'ache all over feeling', and get so tired they 'crash' periodically. On top of all that, their teeth hurt. Doctors tend to chalk it all up to nervous tension, leaving the frustrated patient more confused than ever.

Trouble is these people go to many different doctors for all these pains. So no one doctor hears the whole story. Patients are told it's all in their minds. They are sent to psychiatrists or told to take up a hobby and quit complaining. What a relief it is finally to hear someone say, "Your problems may all be related. There is this little known condition called Sjogren's syndrome." Even though we don't yet have a "cure", there are many ways to treat, or alleviate, the symptoms of SS.

SJOGREN'S SYNDROME: The Sneaky "Arthritis" defines the syndrome and its symptoms; gives a brief history of its identification; covers diagnosis, treatment and prognosis; and discusses the current research and support. All with a dollop of humor. Its goal is to translate complex medical terminology into simple, easy to read language. If it brings comfort and understanding to even one reader this effort will be worthwhile. **You are NOT alone.**
-Sue Dauphin, 1988

FOREWORD

"*Sjogren's Syndrome: the Sneaky "Arthritis"* is an extremely interesting and valuable contribution to the understanding and management of this little understood, or even recognised, disease. It reads easily and in many regards unfolds like a novel, but is, unfortunately, only too true. It should be read by every Sjogren's sufferer as well as by every doctor and dentist. I promise they will benefit by doing so."

Dr. Robert J. Kassan, MD
President, Southeast Florida Arthritis Foundation

"The most common questions asked me by Sjogren's syndrome patients are: "What is Sjogren's syndrome? How can I learn more about this disease?" Referring physicians often ask me for material for their patients with SS. Sjogren's Syndrome Foundation chapters are being formed worldwide. Their newsletter provides a source of information on SS but until now, there has been no book specifically designed for patients.
Sjogren's Syndrome: the Sneaky "Arthritis" by Sue Dauphin is written specifically for SS patients and their families by a professional journalist who has Sjogren's syndrome. The book provides important information on symptoms, treatment, and research. It's style, with a touch of humour, can be understood by the average patient Many physicians may find helpful information and an enhanced understanding of Sjogren's syndrome by reading the book. Being written by a Sjogren's syndrome patient who has experienced, first hand, the frustration of dismissal and delayed diagnosis adds credence to the book's messages.
This book addresses the needs of SS patients and their families for information about this fascinating autoimmune disease. Awareness, cooperation and education form the intelligent approach to understanding and managing this capricious disorder."

Dr. Elaine Alexander, MD
Johns Hopkins University Medical School

Some comments received during research for
Sjogren's Syndrome: the Sneaky Arthritis

"Too few doctors know about this disease. The most important job we have is education; patient education, family education..."
>Dr. Norman Talal, MD
>Chief of Clinical Immunology, University of
>Texas Health Science Center at San Antonio, TX

"I would like to congratulate you for your effort to write a laymen's book for Sjogren's syndrome. It is needed."
>Dr. H. M. Moutsopoulos, MD
>Chairman of Internal Medicine, University
>of Ioannina Medical School, Greece;

"I am impressed by your intention to write a book. I am sure your book will encourage our patients."
>Dr. Susumi Sugai, MD
>Kanazawa Medical University, Japan

"I know fear and what not knowing can do to you. Good luck on your book. It is sorely needed."
>Doris Reprogel, patient, Baltimore MD

"I talked to nurses about SS. None had heard of it. My goal was to increase awareness but I was dealing with my own feelings of isolation, fear, anger."
>Jane Tarail, patient/nurse/writer, San Francisco CA

"I am glad to share my experiences with others."
>Rose Thomas, patient, Chesterland, OH

"Is anything being done on research?"
>Bernice Kapalin, patient, Macedonia, OH

"My doctor's treatment was a 'lube job' in my mouth. I dripped oil. Nothing came of it."
>Helen Ruhl, patient, Detroit MI

Introduction

SJOGREN'S SYNDROME: THE SNEAKY "ARTHRITIS"

Chapter 1

Introduction

"Do you like to eat saltines?"
That simple question was the first in a long series my doctor asked, that led, finally, to a surprise diagnosis. After twenty years of being told I had rheumatoid arthritis (RA), and being treated accordingly, I was sitting in a new rheumatologist's office listening to him describe an ailment I had never heard of.
Sjogren's syndrome, he was telling me, was not actually a single disease, but as its name implies, a collection of symptoms. Symptoms that involved eyes that were always dry, a dry mouth, and the aching joints that inspired the RA diagnosis.

The problems of Sjogren's syndrome are so diverse that they often go unrecognized as having any relation to each other. A patient may, as I did, go to an ophthalmologist for an explanation of blurred vision, a dermatologist about dry and irritated skin, a urologist about recurring infections, and an internist about the aching and swollen joints of arthritis. Dentists and dental technicians constantly admonish her about the build-up of plaque and excessive cavities which seems to go on constantly in spite of ardent brushing and flossing.

No one, least of all the patient, sees any correlation among all these ailments, and more often than not, the patient ignores or suppresses some symptoms for fear of being considered a hypochondriac. In addition, the separate symptoms develop at different rates, and surface (or at least become annoying enough to demand attention) at different times in the patient's lifetime.

Early Symptoms

Although I had always, as long as I can remember, had an aversion to crackers and other dry foods such as the gritty corn bread that is so essential to Southern menus, I never gave it a thought as a medical problem, until the very moment when my doctor asked that deceptively simple question. Different patients report different symptoms as the first sign of trouble. Fabric salesperson Mary Jones'* irritated eyes and blurry vision were laid to the presence of sizing dust in her shop atmosphere. Young Celeste Johnson's mother reacted to Celeste's frequent "swollen glands" by keeping her home from school for a day and giving her chicken soup. Celeste's cousin John claimed to have had "mumps" three times, once more than the medical maximum.

---

* Some names have been changed to protect confidentiality.

Introduction

The author's story begins

In my case the first recognizable sign of trouble was swollen and aching elbows and wrists. I remember very well how it started. I had transplanted a whole hedge of shrubs from an abandoned home down the street to my own yard, digging each one up, lifting it into the trunk of my car and reversing the chore at my home. There were at least 20 of the privet type bushes and I was proud of the effect as they all lined up along the edge of my property. The next day, a Saturday, we went out with friends on their boat. They were enthusiastic water-skiers and urged us to try the sport. My husband was instantly good at it but I was never quite able to get up on my feet with the skis firmly set under me. I tried gamely, a dozen or so times but finally gave up. One reason for my difficulty, which I wouldn't admit to the others, was that my elbows and wrists were hurting more with each try as the tow rope tightened to pull me afloat.

By the following Monday, my knuckles had joined the ranks of the swollen. My aches were severe enough to get me to my family doctor, an internist who gave me an immediate diagnosis. It required only a casual examination of my hands and arms. He noted the bulges on the outer sides of both wrists. "Arthritis," he said. And then because my pain was symmetrical, the same on both sides of my body, he added, "Rheumatoid". So confidant was he of his pronouncement, that he said tests, though available, were not necessary.

Thus began a long series of treatments that included Indocin and massive doses of aspirin. I took these consistently for about 10 years, until I developed an ulcer and was told to discontinue all medication. A hot whirlpool, installed in my home at my doctor's prescription, was to be my only concession to the aching joints from then on.

Different patients, different experiences

Other patients had different experiences but with striking similarities. Janet Walker, an elementary school teacher, traces her problems to a common occupational hazard. Midway through a particularly trying day of math exercises and science labs, she discovered she had broken out in neck-to-toe spots. Only later did one of her students tell her, "That's what Tammy had!" The eighth grader had contracted a rare childhood virus related to the four rashes of the measles family and Janet picked it up from her. Little Tammy's spots were so seldom seen they were known simply as "the fifth rash". Because another teacher at her school was pregnant, Janet stayed home to be on the safe side. The rash was followed within 24 hours by a still more unwelcome set of symptoms. Janet's hands became swollen and tender, making the simplest tasks painful. Her knees became so inflamed, she couldn't walk. Just getting up from a couch was a stressful task. Opening doors was difficult and dressing herself almost impossible.

Although the fifth rash is not a part of Sjogren's syndrome, hindsight indicates that the trauma of the virus may have triggered Janet's later problems. She only knows the aches never quite left her joints and she just didn't rebound to her former springy level of energy. It was also at this time that she began having eye troubles. Like a television screen in an electric storm, Janet's vision was cluttered with blind patches, zig-zag lines and technicolor flashes. Her eyes were scratchy and irritated. Not until many years later was any connection made between her erratic vision and her painful joints.

Twenty-two year old Charles Swenson tells a different story. He recalls going to his South Texas home for Thanksgiving a couple of years back, hoping his mother wouldn't notice the strange puffiness of his cheeks. Mother did notice, of course, and insisted he see a doctor. Charles didn't want to admit to his parents and his nine brothers and sisters that he, too, was a

Introduction

little concerned. The swellings along his jaws had been coming and going for some time for no apparent reason. Friends commented that he had gained (or lost) weight, according to whether his jaws were swollen or not on any given day. He had had mumps as a boy, so he and his mother could only think some kind of infection was behind his chipmunk-like appearance. The holiday over, he went back to his college and set up an appointment with a local general practitioner. The doctor prescribed medication for the sore throat that also bothered Charles, but was hard put to explain the swollen glands. It seemed that something might be blocking the passages. The soreness of Charles' throat subsided, but the puffy pouches remained.

After about four months, Charles sought out another doctor who at once suspected Sjogren's syndrome. Although tests gave mixed results, the doctor felt the diagnosis was confirmed and recommended surgery to remove Charles' defective saliva glands. The young student was understandably hesitant about such a drastic step and sought another opinion. This time the testing was extensive and conclusive. He did indeed have Sjogren's syndrome but the new doctors were reluctant to operate, suggesting he postpone that as long as possible. There were ways to deal with his dry mouth in the meantime. He discovered that the red eyes he had been blaming on too much late night studying, were really part of the syndrome and could also be treated. At least Charles now had a diagnosis. He could begin to cope. Coping was becoming increasingly difficult for Betty Rosen, a suburban wife, mother of three and caregiver for her husband's elderly parents, who were victims of Parkinson's and Alzheimer's diseases. This shouldn't have been too much for her to handle, but she was constantly tired and a variety of problems plagued her. Her eyes became too irritated to tolerate the contact lenses she tried to wear. She repeatedly lost her voice for no apparent reason.

The tiredness progressed to weakness and a "hurt all over feeling". She began using a cane to help her walk. This struck her as unreasonable, since she

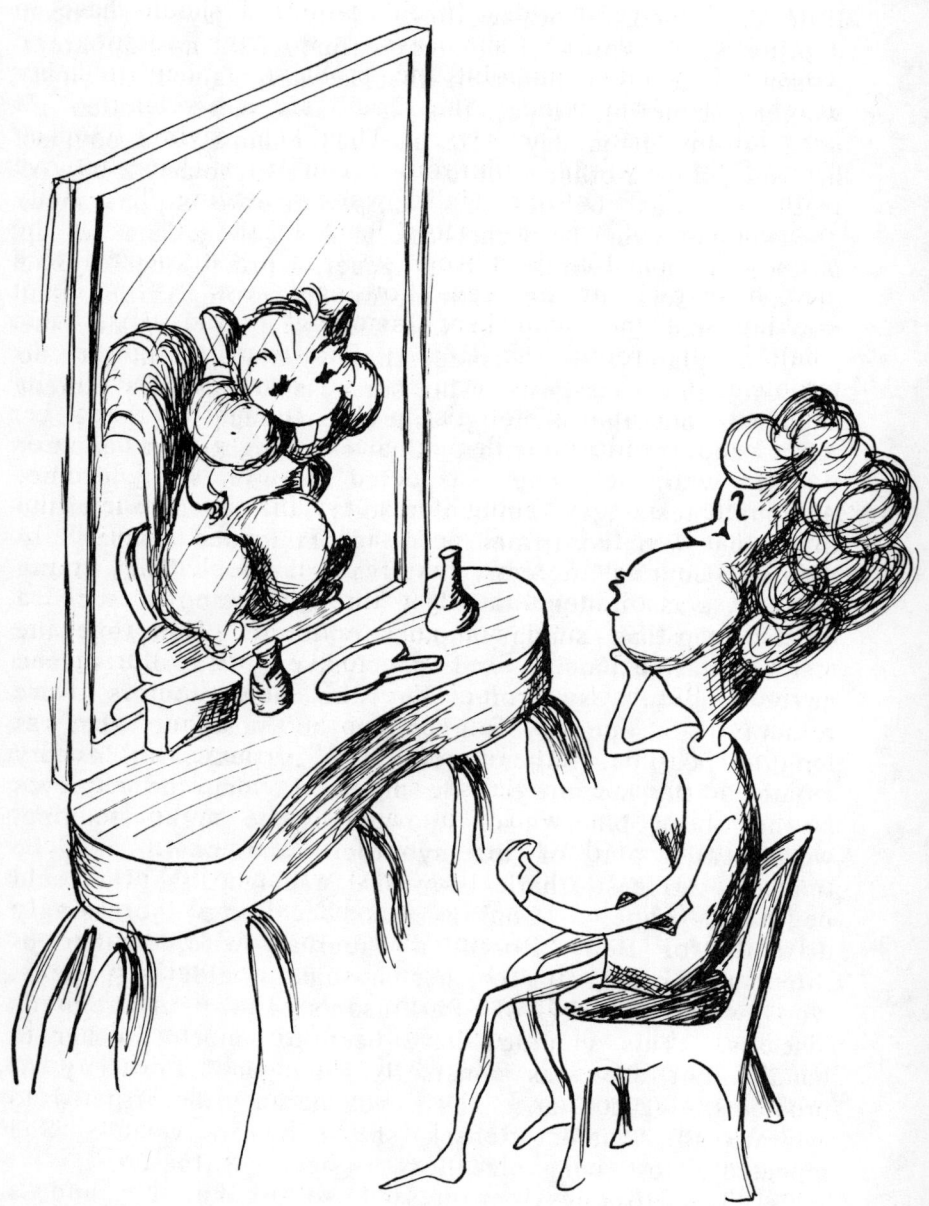

Figure 1   Cheeks Like a Chipmunk

Introduction

was only 30 years old. "I didn't think I should have to use a cane at 30." she says. But the doctors she consulted couldn't pinpoint the problem. They told her it was all in her mind. She should see a psychiatrist. "I was falling apart", she says. "They kept saying 'I can't find a thing wrong with you. You'll just have to live with it.'" Then one night, while watching TV, Betty happened to glance at a table lamp in the corner of the room. It looked as if it were smoking. She checked with her husband but he saw nothing amiss. She kept looking and the lamp kept "smoking" And there were "halos" all around the light. She tried to ignore the problem but the halos wouldn't go away so she finally went to an ophthalmologist. He thought perhaps her eyes were prematurely aging, but could give no reason for it.

Betty did try going to a psychiatrist. She stuck with that for five years and says it helped emotionally, but did nothing to solve her physical problems. Prayer, she says, also helped her get through these times. But the halos still would not go away and walking became even more difficult. She went to 19 doctors during this period. But each one looked at a different aspect of her situation. In a familiar pattern, she saw an ophthalmologist, an internist, an orthopedist, and a bone and muscle specialist, among others. Finally, she saw an internist who took a different approach. He made it a challenge to identify her problem. Betty wrote down everything that was wrong with her. The list covered "a huge page and it was tiny, tiny handwriting." The doctor came to the conclusion she had lupus, or if not, some other connective tissue disease. Her blood tests were always just a slightly off the norm but not enough so to make a firm diagnosis. Things came to a head when she began falling down with no warning. "I'd just topple over as if someone had turned my key off." The internist sent Betty to a muscle specialist who, familiar with Sjogren's syndrome, was able finally to connect all the dots in Betty's clinical records. He told her she had Sjogren's syndrome, secondary to dermatomyositis, the form of connective tissue disease that attacks muscles. The extraordinary weakness of Betty's legs was at last explained and she was able to begin treatment. For Betty Rosen, the road to diagnosis had taken six years.

My journey was longer, perhaps because it began earlier when the awareness of Sjogren's syndrome was even less widespread than it is now. With treatment, my ulcer healed, but the aching of the joints persisted. I faithfully continued to take two baths per day in my hot tub. The fact that my skin became progressively drier seemed only a small price to be paid for the soothing effects of the baths. But those effects were short-lived and the pain would inevitably return soon after the towel finished its work. What's more, new problems appeared. Knees, hips and back chimed in to let me know all was not well. When I complained to my doctor, he told me I would simply have to choose between putting up with my aches, or ruining my stomach.

About that time I decided to look elsewhere for medical care. My new doctor, a general practitioner, helped me begin a search for a suitable treatment, using an NSAID (Non-Steroidal Anti-Inflammatory Drug). The list of drugs we tried would read like a pharmacist's order list. They came in all sizes and shapes. Round blue pills. Green and white capsules. Huge oval tablets. Fortunately, there is a wide assortment of these anti-inflammatory agents to choose from. Most arthritis patients are familiar with them through this same process of selection to find the one that is effective for them. It would seem at first that I was tolerating the drug, and the relief from the pains was indeed pleasant. But soon the familiar burning sensation would begin in my stomach and I would know that that particular drug was not for me.

Meanwhile, I saw several eye doctors about the blurry mucus I couldn't seem to clear out of my eyes. And I suffered increasing allergic reactions to multiple or unidentified substances. After one particularly severe session which was blamed on one of the NSAID's I tried, I was started on the corticosteroid, Prednisone.

Introduction

When my rash subsided I cut way down but continued a low dosage of the popular cortisone drug. A later skin rash brought me to an allergist who expressed dismay at my long-term use of cortisone and told me some of the possible side effects I had not known about. (The side effects of cortisone and other drugs will be discussed in Chapter 5.) It was this concern that finally inspired me to seek out the specialized help of the rheumatologist who finally labeled my Sjogren's syndrome.

Sjogren's Syndrome Defined

What do all these patients have in common? A lot of things. But the thing that stands out most sharply in all the stories is the multiplicity of their symptoms and the resulting difficulty of diagnosis. The problems they have stem from the fact that the disease has long been considered rare and until recently was given short shrift in medical schools. A doctor in his 40s or older would probably have heard Sjogren's mentioned only briefly during his student days. He was probably told that he was not likely to see actual cases during his regular practice. Younger doctors now training receive much more information and are therefore more aware of it, especially in those disciplines affected by the syndrome. Thus it is still possible, in fact researchers think much more common than is known, for patients to go to many doctors who, quite innocently, fail to correlate the symptoms described. Additionally, because of the overlapping nature of many of Sjogren's symptoms, it is often hard to distinguish between Sjogren's and rheumatoid arthritis or lupus. According to Dr. Frank Arnett, Director of the Rheumatology Division of the University of Texas Health Science Center in Houston. and a leading Sjogren's researcher, "The borders are blurred, even for the experts. We have pretty well separated RA and Sjogren's but lupus is more difficult. The serious research into SS has only really begun in the '80s."

The common symptoms, those necessary for a

clinical diagnosis of Sjogren's syndrome, as my doctor informed me, are dry eyes, dry mouth, and aching joints. Any two of these are enough to qualify a patient as having Sjogren's syndrome. In this simple form, it is known as Primary Sjogren's syndrome. This means Sjogren's syndrome without one of an assortment of the connective tissue diseases, such as rheumatoid arthritis, which often accompany it. Others include SLE (systemic lupus erythematosus or lupus), scleroderma, polymyositis, and dermatomyositis, All of these are disorders that occur when the body's immune system turns against us. Cells in the blood stream, which are designed to protect us from invading germs and disease organisms, become "confused" and attack our own tissues, instead of the enemy. The type of cells doing the attacking and of tissue under siege defines the disease. In the case of Sjogren's syndrome, the body's exocrine glands, particularly the tear glands and the salivary glands, are the victims of marauding cells from the bloodstream which invade the glands and prevent them from producing the fluids that lubricate the eyes or mouth. As is obvious from our case stories, other organs can be and usually are involved. These, as well as the related connective tissue diseases of secondary Sjogren's syndrome, their treatment, and the outlook for the future will be discussed further in later chapters. From the ranks of the fairly recently formed Sjogren's Syndrome Foundation's chapters all over the country I have gleaned many tales of the great variety of manifestations of the disease. I will quote from these experiences throughout the book to illustrate the problems encountered by typical SS victims. I don't want to add to the worries of those who might have Sjogren's syndrome, but to increase the general awareness of the condition so many more people may identify the source of their annoying problems, and begin, as our cases have, to cope. And to let the people involved know they are definitely not alone.

Introduction

A chronic autoimmune disease

Sjogren's syndrome is a chronic autoimmune disease in which the immune system, the body's network of defense mechanisms, reacts against itself. A certain type of lymphocyte, a white blood corpuscle which circulates in the blood and lymph systems, normally mobilizes to fight off infections and foreign bodies. They produce the antibodies that give us immunity to diseases once conquered, such as measles. But sometimes some of these cells turn against the very body they are supposed to protect. They infiltrate and damage exocrine(mucus-secreting) glands as if they were foreign bodies. The injured glands are no longer able to lubricate our mouths, eyes, joints, and other parts of our bodies.

Secondary SS

When the familiar triad of symptoms is present along with one of several connective tissue diseases, it is considered secondary Sjogren's syndrome. Probably as many as half of all people with rheumatoid arthritis also have Sjogren's syndrome. They are most often the ones who don't know of their SS because the arthritis symptoms are much more demanding of attention. In fact, it might be 40 years from the time RA is diagnosed to the time the first symptoms of Sjogren's syndrome are recognized.

Some surprising numbers

For many years Sjogren's syndrome has been considered a rare disease, but doctors and researchers are becoming more and more convinced it has been seriously underrated. However, because of the lack of documented cases, and because so many people go undiagnosed, there is great confusion, even among the experts, as to how common the disease really is. As early as 1971, writing in his book *Sjogren's Syndrome*, M. A. Shearn [70] estimated that SS "affects an estimated

2% of the population." He pointed out that "the frequency with which it is recognized depends in large measure on the frame of reference and the awareness of the physician who initially sees the patient." He mentions a patient who had been seen 22 times by ophthalmologists for "chronic conjunctivitis" before anyone thought of SS. Various doctors have made educated guesses based on the number of rheumatoid arthritis patients they have seen who also have KCS (keratoconjunctivitis sicca). Naturally, this brings differing results, but the number of RA patients who also have SS ranges from 30 to 50 percent. Dr. Norman Talal, writing for *Drug Therapy*[75] in 1984 calculates that if 25 percent of the nation's 8 million Rheumatoid patients have SS and an equal number have SS without RA, there must be at least 4 million SS sufferers, many as yet undetected. Another statistic says that every year, a million people will be told for the first time that they have arthritis. How many of those will have SS along with or instead of their arthritis is almost impossible to guess, but estimates say 30 to 50% of SS patients also have RA; 5 to 8%, scleroderma; 4 to 5%, lupus.

Probably second only to RA in frequency, SS is found among men and women of all ages, but ninety percent of patients are women, usually middle aged and white. Still, studies have been made of groups of children with SS, even as young as two and a half years old.[20] The disease for them turned out to be similar to that of the adults. This also proved true when comparisons were made between men and women patients. No significant differences were noted in age, racial distribution, onset, and length of disease or symptoms, except that men were more likely to have extra complications as opposed to the glandular syndrome alone. Differences noted in blood chemistry have led investigators to look into a possible connection of sex hormones similar to that seen in SLE.[52] In considering the occurrence of SS in children, and the long lead time for diagnosis in some cases, it's

Introduction

interesting that many adults, once they have been diagnosed as having SS, will remember details from their younger years that seem to fit right in. Rose Thomas says, "My husband reminds me that I have had various symptoms for many years prior to the 1982 visits to the doctor." Another correspondent told me she had lost all her teeth at age 22. With some surprise, she wondered if that loss could have been connected with SS. Some may have other problems such as chronic thyroid, kidney, or liver conditions. One older patient remembers having irritated eyes all through his school years. The mean time lag between the actual beginnings of the disease and its identification is eight years, but many, as we have seen, go twenty years or longer in the dark as to the real nature of their illness. This book is intended to help avoid that for as many of those people as possible. And to help us get a fix on what Sjogren's syndrome is all about.

In these days of trillion dollar deficits and billion dollar lawsuits, it is becoming increasingly difficult to grasp the significance of statistics such as those I've been quoting. We can gleefully mimic Carl Sagan with his 'billyuns and billyuns' of stars, but we can only see an infinitesimal part of them. I once read that the human brain can deal with only five units at a time. After that we must start making notes. Or counting on our fingers.

To make it easier for us to understand the scope of SS, I'm going to dream up a mythical city with a population of 50 thousand. That's a more manageable number to handle. We'll call it Sicca City and, if you'll forgive me, locate it in the state of Poor Health. Of the 50 thousand men, women and children who live there, we can guess that one thousand will have Sjogren's syndrome. Nine hundred of them are women. Approximately 390 of them also have rheumatoid arthritis, 60 have scleroderma, 40 have lupus, and and a few have other connective tissue diseases like dermatomyositis, polymyositis The remaining 5 hundred have SS alone (primary Sjogren's syndrome.) We'll follow along with our Sicca Citians as we consider all the aspects of SS, and try by that means, to keep it all in perspective.

Chapter 2

Symptoms

Primary Sjogren's Syndrome (Sicca complex)

Once you are diagnosed as having Sjogren's syndrome, your doctor will probably put you into one of Sjogren's two distinct groups. He will say you have Primary Sjogren's syndrome or Secondary Sjogren's syndrome. This will depend on whether you also have one of the rheumatic diseases. If you have dry eyes, dry mouth, and joint pains; or any two of these without any rheumatic diseases (rheumatoid arthritis, lupus, etc.), you have primary Sjogren's syndrome. It is often referred to as sicca complex. "Sicca", which comes from the Latin word siccus (dry), refers to the fact that dryness is the most obvious symptom. There are some significant differences between the two levels of the syndrome, which will be discussed at the end of this chapter.

Dry Eyes (Keratoconjunctivitis)

Actually the first thing you might notice about your eyes could be the kind of thick, gooey secretion that bothered me. It floats annoyingly around in your eyes. Your vision is obscured and you can't quite wipe the mess away. But its an intermittent nuisance that will go away all on it's own after a while and seems always to be gone when you tell your ophthalmologist about it. "How can I tell you what it is when I see nothing there?" is a common reaction. This gooeyness, surprisingly, can be the result of the lack of tears as the glands try to compensate. All of our five hundred Sicca Citians with primary SS have dry eyes and most of the secondary patients do too, as this, along with the dry mouth, is the hallmark of SS.

In Sjogren's syndrome, white blood cells

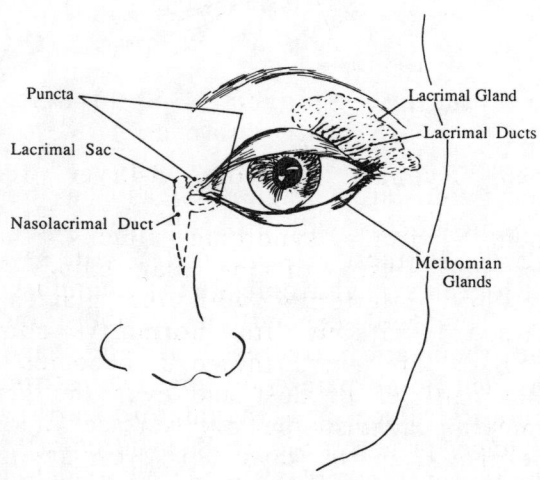

Figure 2 Tear Ducts and Glands

Symptoms

(lymphocytes) invade the tear glands above and outside the eye (lacrimal) and the smaller glands (meibomian) at the edge of the eyelid.

The glands produce the thin, oily outermost layer of the tear film while the watery tears we are familiar with are secreted by the lacrimal gland. Still another layer lies closest to the eyeball. This one is made up of mucus and helps spread the tears evenly over the eye as well as serving as a kind of glue to hold all that moisture in. 9

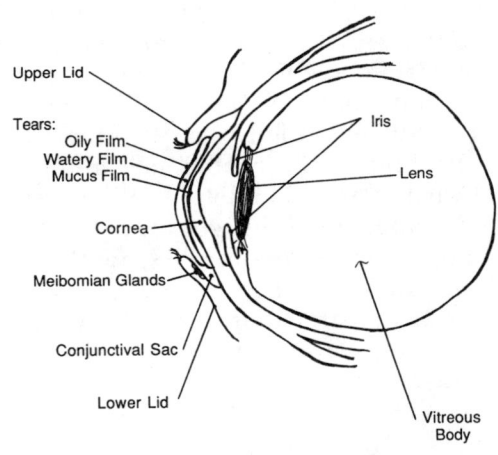

Figure 3 Eyeball showing 3-layer tear film

When Sjogren's syndrome attacks, the invading cells cause the tissue of the tear glands to become fibery and dry, interfering with the gland's ability to make tears. Without its normally soothing and protective bath of tears, the eye becomes subject to assault from particles of dust and even the grating of its own lid moving against the dry surface of the eyeball. Ohioan Bernice Kapalin says her eyes are so dry she "can HEAR them opening and closing." Depending on the amount of damage to the gland, the eye marshals what's left of its ability to protect itself and a filmy blurriness occurs. This comes from the build-up of an abnormal type of mucus that works "like an oil spot on a car's windshield." The watery tears that are still available will not cling over the mucus and vision is obstructed.[40] Other complaints include grittiness, a scratchy feeling, or the sensation of something foreign in the eye. Certain patients have written that they have been bothered with protein deposits on contacts and the appearance of halos around street lights. Keratoconjunctivitis, as it is known medically, also shows up as redness, burning, itching, and extra sensitivity to light (photosensitivity). The eyes feel tired and vision may be less sharp than normal. Since emotional tears are a different sort from these protective ones, the ability to cry from sadness or anger may or may not be affected. The wearing of contact lenses may be ruled out by the irritation. The dryness may be more noticeable at night because our lids do not always close completely while we sleep. The doctors call this *nocturnal lagothpthalmos*. To top that off, actual tear production may slow down at night. Often these symptoms are not severe, causing more of a nuisance and discomfort than any real disability, but without proper care, more-serious problems can follow. The most likely and obvious consequence of the shortage of tears is corneal abrasion, or scratching. Irritation of the blood vessels (vasculitis) is possible as is clouding of the cornea (opacity).[85,75]

Having started this book telling the experiences of two SS patients who experienced flashes and 'zig-zags' of light that disturbed their vision, it is important to discuss these problems here. The normal aging process involves shrinkage of the gelatin-like substance (vitreous humor) that fills the inside of the eyeball. Many of us, at any age, have 'seen' specks or bits of 'debris' that appear to float in front of our eyes. Actually they are inside our eyes, in the vitreous humor. Called floaters they are small clumps of the gel itself and have an annoying way of drifting off when we try to look at them. This is because they are just off center and move with the eye as we try to focus.

Symptoms

Annoying as they may be, these floaters are unimportant and may safely be ignored. If floaters get in the way of whatever you are trying to see, the American Academy of Ophthalmology suggests you move your eye around, looking quickly up and down to 'shake' the floaters into a different position. As we grow older, a much more disturbing thing can happen. We may suddenly see many new floaters at once or flashes of light that persist with no relation to the actual light around us. Although these too, are probably normal changes as part of the aging process, a visit to the ophthalmologist is in order. The lights are most likely the result of minor tears in the retina as the shrinking gel pulls away from it. They will disappear in about a month. But it's possible that a retinal detachment could occur and it is also possible, though apparently uncommon, that the flashes could be caused by inflammation, our old nemesis of SS. For this reason an examination by an ophthalmologist is essential to make sure the problem *is* minor. [8]

Dry Mouth (Xerostomia)

The second major symptom of Sjogren's syndrome is a dry mouth. Again, it is caused by the lymphocytes attacking their own host, your body. This time their target is the salivary glands, those that supply you with saliva. They become tough and stringy, and unable to generate enough saliva to moisten your mouth. This causes an assortment of uncomfortable problems. The most noticeable, perhaps is that, with little or no lubrication of the teeth and gums, things stick to them. Food attaches itself to your teeth and refuses to slide away as it should. Ordinary chewing gum and chewy candies are likely to be the first things you'll eliminate from your diet just because they're too much trouble to eat. The fact that they are especially harmful to the Sjogren's syndrome patient will be discussed later. Lettuce, while healthy for the diet, has a distressing tendency to cling to the teeth. Here's where the question of saltines and bread becomes important. They not only stick to your molars, but they give you trouble all the way down, forming dry lumps that are hard to swallow. One doctor in Mexico, Dr. Guillermo J. Ruiz-Arguelles, even suggests that tell-tale lipstick smears on the teeth be taken as a warning that the possibility that the patient may have Sjogren's syndrome should be investigated. [66]

"Rampant" Tooth Decay

But there is a serious side to this effect. Normally saliva serves as a protective coating for the teeth. It contains ingredients that limit the growth of the bacteria that cause tooth decay at the same time that it bathes the teeth in protective minerals such as calcium, phosphorus, and fluoride. [59] This remineralizes them, replacing lost traces of these essential minerals. Of course, it is obvious that the flow of saliva over the surfaces of the teeth helps to keep them clean, washing away the food particles in between brushings. When this marvelous fluid is in short supply, or missing entirely, its easy to see what the consequences can be. Food scraps do not get washed away and, in fact, bits and pieces of that mid-afternoon snack adhere firmly. Bacteria have a field day, growing at their own, unrestricted pace. The reservoir of minerals (calcium, phosphorus and fluoride), is depleted and not available for the day-to-day healing the average person enjoys. The teeth are left defenseless against the assaults of acids in such foods as citrus fruits.

The infamous plaque that television advertisements warn us against builds up rapidly. It contains more bacteria and is harder to remove. Cavities abound and your teeth are in real danger from decay. My husband used to complain that I had "teeth like butter." The world said I had a "sweet tooth" and ate too much candy. So aside from all the pain of toothaches, and the inconvenience of frequent trips to the dentist, the Sjogren's syndrome victim lives with guilty feelings that the dental problems are all his or

Symptoms

her fault. I preferred to blame my troubles on an early dentist who discouraged my mother from having my teeth straightened with braces when I was a child. In those days the straightening would have cost $300 and he told her it wasn't worth it. Now, just capping one of those crooked teeth costs more than that. But poor, long abused Dr. Weston no longer must bear all the blame for my decimated teeth.

Thirst and Throat Problems

The dryness caused by lack of saliva extends, naturally, beyond just its effects on the teeth. The entire mouth needs lubrication and doesn't get it. Factors in the saliva meant to lubricate food are missing. The enzymes that should be in the saliva to start dissolving the food and give the digestive process a boost are decreased or not there at all. The result is difficulty in swallowing. You feel the sensation of a lump in your throat that can even be painful at times and the discomfort can go all the way down the esophagus as the food passes through. [41] On top of that, the soft tissues of the mouth are dry, making you thirsty much of the time. Sara Endress had the frightening experience of waking up in the middle of the night, with a choking sensation as if her throat was totally closed. The surface of the tongue may be irritated, split, and sensitive to heat, cold, and peppery foods. Lips and corners of the mouth may crack and be sore and there may be ulcers inside the mouth. All these problems leave your mouth susceptible to infections. The dryness provides a particularly favorable climate for yeast infections (most commonly Candidiasis) to grow. [68] To add insult to injury, the ability to enjoy the taste of sweet, sour, salty, or bitter foods can be diminished, although some of us who have diet problems might consider that a blessing! Apparently the reduction in saliva brings about a corresponding reduction in the number of taste buds, and then makes matters worse by dampening the tasting ability of the ones that are left. 33

As Sjogren's syndrome is an inflammatory process, a painful swelling of the affected glands is all too often a part of the syndrome. In particular, the parotid glands around the mouth may become enlarged. About half of all Sjogren's syndrome patients have parotid glands that swell repeatedly as Charles Swenson's did. That's about 500 from our Sicca City group, anywhere from 250 to 400 of them primary SS patients. The jaws may puff out separately or both at the same time, and feel tender, red, and feverish. It can happen suddenly and subside just as swiftly. They seldom become infected, but a hard or lumpy gland could signify a tumor and should be investigated. Helen

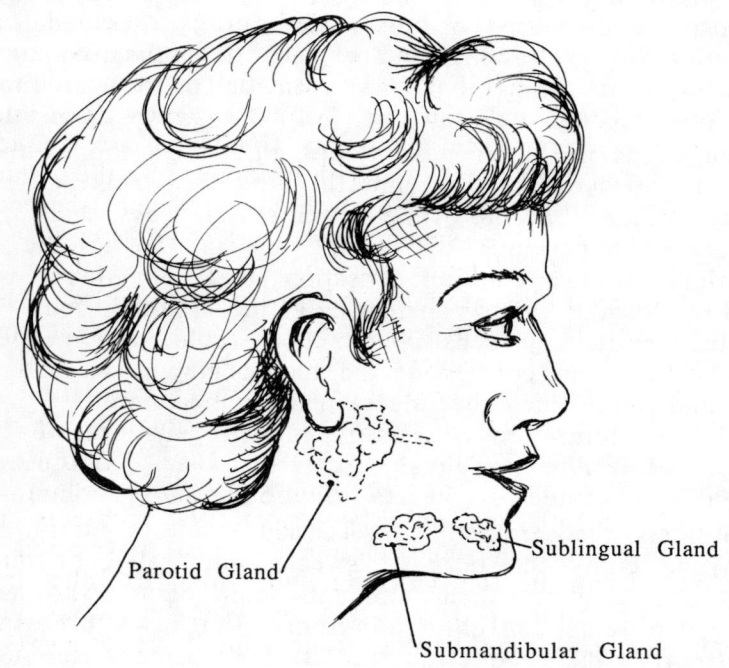

Figure 4 Salivary Glands 16

Symptoms

Ruhl of Detroit, says her swollen cheeks that made her look like a kewpie doll were the first symptom that sent her looking for medical help.

If all this is beginning to sound terribly uncomfortable, remember that few people have all these symptoms at once, and some of them never. And keep reading; we will discuss the ways of alleviating the ones you do have.

Joint Pain

The painful joints and morning stiffness so similar to the key symptoms of rheumatoid arthritis (RA) are partly responsible for the frequent mix-ups in diagnosis. But, in a rare piece of good news for Sjogren's syndrome sufferers, the pain and inflammation of primary Sjogren's syndrome is usually mild and seldom results in the deformities expected with RA. And, if you are going to have secondary Sjogren's syndrome, you usually get the associated tissue disease (RA, etc.) first, and the SS symptoms show up later. Thus, if you have sicca symptoms first, you are unlikely to develop the RA later. With primary SS, the joints most often hurting are the small ones, and the pain comes and goes. It is symmetrical as it is in RA; that is, it will usually affect both sides of the body at the same time. Aileen Lull's troubles began in her ankles. Her doctor called it 'sprains' and sent her to a psychiatrist when she refused to accept that.

If your right wrist hurts, chances are the left one does, too. When the right knee complains, the left knee is heard from at the same time. The joints may be swollen and warm. The inflammation occurs when the lubricating sheath (synovial capsule) that protects the joint is dried up and non-functional. You may often be stiff first thing in the morning, but this generally lasts only a short time. If you get up and go about your normal business, the stiffness will usually fade away in a half hour or so.

Other Exocrine Glands

The glands of the eyes and mouth (tear glands and salivary glands) are part of a system designed to lubricate the various organs throughout the body. Known as exocrine glands, they secrete fluids [57] or mucus to cushion the friction of tissue upon tissue or smooth the way for a particular organ to carry out its appointed function. Exocrine glands are also found in the nasal passages, the lower respiratory system, the digestive tract, the vaginal area, and the skin.

The Lower Respiratory System

Mucous glands line the walls of the larynx (voice box), and the esophagus (the tubes that carry food to the stomach and air to the lungs). When Sjogren's syndrome dries up these glands, hoarseness. can result, along with a feeling of constant congestion, of needing to clear the throat. A dry cough can develop as well as frequent sore throats. The dryness here as well as in the mouth can, in severe cases, make speech difficult. Speaking for long periods, or singing, can put stress on a dry throat and vocal cords.

An irritation of the lining of the lungs (pleurisy) makes the chest sore, but some researchers claims this occurs infrequently. Bronchitis, shortness of breath, [22] and pneumonia are also possibilities, but there is controversy in the medical world as to how closely related these symptoms are to SS. [7,18,21,62,73] Kathy Marsh moved south to Houston to avoid the hard winters that seemed to be making her ill, and later, suddenly and unexpectedly became desperately ill with pneumonia. Intensive care and a month's hospitalization pulled her through that but she had two recurrences. Even after her complaints about her dry mouth finally turned up a diagnosis of SS, her doctors disagree as to whether the pneumonia is a function of the Sjogren's.

Symptoms

Nasal Passages and Ears

Similarly, mucous membranes in the nasal passages may dry up, causing burning or itching (rhinitis). Irritations can lead to nosebleeds that seem to happen just to spite you. And, as in the eyes, compensatory efforts by the struggling glands can bring on the stuffiness of congestion. The same process that robs some of their tasting abilities, is also at work here, interfering with the sense of smell.[33] The pathways (eustachian tubes) between the middle ear and the throat can be affected causing inflammation and a (generally) slight loss of hearing. Sara Endress reports, after years of eye and throat problems, that her ears are beginning to hurt, especially when in a draft from air conditioning. She finds putting cotton in them provides some protection. Sara lives in Arizona and uses a 'swamp cooler', a unit that adds moisture to the air it cools, instead of drying it as does an air conditioner. Now we are beginning to get an idea what is meant by "that ache all over feeling."

Vaginal Dryness

One of those problems many women are reluctant to discuss with their doctors is vaginal dryness. Or if they do complain to a gynecologist, they are often treated for recurring infections. Or if no infection is found, "vaginitis" is the diagnosis and we are told to ignore it and it will go away.

There are many causes of vaginal dryness. Dr. Thomas Sheehy, Jr. lists several, including excess use of soap, douches, or bath powder.[71] Even plain tap water can be the culprit. Soap, even mild soap, contains lye which is caustic. Prepared douches contain perfumes and dyes. Bath powder just naturally soaks up moisture. But tap water? Even the purest contains chemicals as well as traces of metal it picks up on its way through the plumbing pipes. The menstrual cycle, its ending, and changing hormone levels all have their effects.

And, for once, it may actually be 'all in your mind.' Stress, fatigue, and an emotional upset can interfere with vaginal lubrication. Dryness can go along with 'Not tonight, dear, I have a headache.'

But for SS patients, it's the old story of glands that fail to function. There are two of them, called Bartholin's glands, located in the walls of the vagina, whose purpose is lubrication. As in other glands, lymphocytic infiltration can disrupt the ability to secrete the necessary fluids. And remember how our other beleaguered glands try hard to make up for the lack of their proper fluids? These are no exception and the resulting mucous discharges mimic infections. Dryness and irritation invite frequent real infections, and it has been speculated, the treatment for these can create a vicious cycle by causing more irritation. The lack of moisture can also bring pain to intercourse.

Don't be too distressed by all this. Ways to prevent and/or alleviate these problems are discussed in the chapter on treatment.

Dry skin

For some, a most annoying symptom is a dryness of the skin. The wrinkles that come with it make the skin look prematurely aged. Sjogren's syndrome patients also bruise easily. They may have rashes that hang around longer than ordinary hives would, small lumps (nodules) just under the skin, or sores and cracks. Purple marks (purpura) made by tiny broken and inflamed blood vessels (vasculitis) directly under the skin especially on the legs, may leave a brown coloring from iron deposits remaining after the bruise has faded. The surface of the skin may have small depressions from loss of fat under the skin, or nodules that appear as small lumpy spots under the skin. [5,6] Bernice Kapalin complains that at 55, this loss of fat cells has made her look 'a lot older' than she is. SS patients do not sweat as easily, which may seem to the fastidious to be a plus, until we remember that perspiration serves to cool and cleanse the skin.

Symptoms

Another dimension added to the dry skin problem is a dry scalp and with it, dry hair.

While most of these skin problems are mere annoyances, it is important to note that the surface vasculitis, indicated by chronic hives or those purple marks on your legs, could be an indication of a more serious vasculitis going on in internal parts of your body. Vasculitis can impair the function of the gastrointestinal system, muscles, or the central nervous system (brain and spinal column). While this is relatively rare, the appearance of these outward markers should be a sign to investigate and eliminate the possiblilty of potential danger. This is an area where the condition is treatable and early diagnosis can help avoid trouble.

Extraglandular Symptoms

But hold on. There's more. Other complications vary considerably with each person. About one-fourth of the patients with primary Sjogren's syndrome have one or more of the following problems. Thus in our mythical Sicca City, with its 1000 Sjogren's syndrome patients, 250 fall into this category.

The blood vessels, spleen, liver, pancreas, muscles, and thyroid can all get into the act.[75] They, too, may become irritated and inflamed. About 150 of our Sicca City friends may have kidney problems. In addition, the digestive system and the central and peripheral nervous systems sometimes get involved.

Raynaud's phenomenon is a name given to the situation where the fingers become very sensitive to cold, heat, or emotional stress. They become white, then blue, and may be numb or tingle and burn briefly before returning to normal.[13] At least one of my correspondents has complained that her feet are always cold.

The excessive need to urinate often comes as a side effect of the dry mouth that inspires a constant thirst and, consequently, continual drinking of fluids.

Under normal circumstances our kidneys are assigned the task of excreting wastes and regulating the body's water, electrolyte and acid/base balance. This is accomplished, in part, by recycling the excess water we take in. In rare cases the marauding lymphocytes of Sjogren's syndrome inhibit that recycling ability. A short supply of anti-diuretic hormones interferes with the kidneys' perception of water quantity. They simply excrete water, whether excess or not. As the body's water level goes down, the concentration of electrolytes goes up and the balance is disturbed. However, this happens extremely seldom and even then is usually so slight that you're not likely to notice it and you should not be worried about it. Chances are, if you need to urinate often, it's because you are drinking a lot of fluids. This also results in a need to get up several times during the night. Irritation of the lining of the bladder (interstitial cystitis)[4,5] makes this problem worse when the bladder's walls swell and restrict its capacity. This is another one that often doesn't come to the attention of the rheumatologist. Your family doctor will refer you to a urologist who, quite naturally, will not be particularly concerned with the condition of your eyes and mouth.

Digestive System

Acid secreting glands in the stomach and mucous glands in the intestines become lazy and fail to do their jobs. Result? Poor digestion and unspecific pains that resist identification. Here there can be even more reason for confusion. By this time your doctor has surely prescribed some anti-inflammatory drugs, such as aspirin or ibuprofen. They are the ones subject to the big TV commercial advertising campaigns based on the claims that they will not upset your stomach. Sometimes they do cause stomach problems for some people. They are even said to be responsible for the formation of ulcers, but how are we to know whether it

Symptoms

is the pills or the illness that is causing the trouble? [87] According to Dr. Adolf Van Mulders and his associates, Sjogren's syndrome rather than the drugs may be the culprit.

The digestive process begins in the mouth when we chew our food. From that point on a series of mechanical and chemical steps break down the food for the body's use. Enzymes in the saliva initiate the action as the food passes quickly through the mouth and is carried down to the stomach. There, gastric glands secrete more enzymes, hydrochloric acid, and mucus, which combine to continue the process. Moving right along, the food (by now known as chyme) passes into the upper part of the intestine (the duodenum). More glands secrete digestive juice from the pancreas to further convert the chyme. Digestion continues as the food elements are absorbed into the bloodstream and the residues are processed and moved out of the body. From this brief account it is easy to see how anything that interferes with the action of all these glands can disrupt the whole digestive process. My correspondents complain variously of choking on dry food, of indigestion, abdominal pain, gas, constipation, diarrhea, nausea, diverticulitis, ulcers, frequent urination and bladder problems, although, admittedly, some of these may be only indirectly related to Sjogren's, if at all. We do have to use restraint in the tendency to blame EVERYTHING on the SS.

From childhood I have had a digestive system that didn't follow the rules. For me, an apple a day did not keep the doctor away. In fact, apples and all those other high-fiber foods that are so popular now, aggravated the constipation that seemed always lurking, ready to plague me. It still does. And a high fiber, low-fat diet makes it worse. Only recently has it occurred to me to speculate about that relationship. Especially when I read that the way fiber helps is by absorbing moisture from the intestines, thus expanding and creating beneficial bulk. But we have learned that the SS patient is likely to have inefficient glands secreting insufficient digestive juices. Why wouldn't the thirsty fiber soak it all up and still be left too dry?

Dr. Seymour Katz of the Long Island Jewish Medical Center lists some other problems that can be caused or complicated by SS.[39] Some patients have trouble with 'webs', the narrowing of the lowermost cartilage of the larynx, called 'cricoid' because of its shape, resembling a signet ring. These can cause difficulty in swallowing and may or may not be related to SS. The muscles of the esophagus may not contract properly, and thus may also be causing that swallowing problem as well as heartburn (acid rising from the stomach or refluxing), and chest pain that can frighten you into thinking you are having angina. Sometimes, especially in children, the lower end of the esophagus tenses (achalasia) and won't let food pass through smoothly.

I would suspect the most common problem would be gastritis, plain old nagging 'tummy ache' that comes from a lack of acid, rather than the familiar "excess acidity" the advertisers love to tout. In this case the pain, a burning sensation, and, for some people, nausea, is due to irritation of the stomach lining. Doctors call this shortage of digestive acids "achlorhydria."

More serious situations can involve and inflammation of the pancreas (pancreatitis), the liver (chronic active hepatitis), cirrhosis or inflammatory bowel disease, but Dr.Katz hastens to remind us that in mentioning these and a few other complications we should note that they are relatively rare in proportion to the overall number of Sjogren's patients. Especially since the ones the gastroenterologist sees are only those who already have intestinal problems. "Although your chances of having one of these GI diseases may be somewhat higher than those of someone without Sjogren's syndrome," he says, "your likelihood is still quite small."

Central and Peripheral Nervous Systems

Less obvious is the relationship of the central nervous system to SS but studies have shown that certain problems do occur. Included are mild memory lapses (who among us has not had an occasion to forget our best friend's name just when we need to introduce him to someone?); difficulties in concentration (and we thought that was just because the children were screaming at us!); and mild mood swings from excitement to depression. Some patients find they have less sensitivity to touch. Their fingers or toes may tingle, prickle or just feel numb.[38] Some patients are afflicted with carpal tunnel syndrome, a tenderness and weakness of the thumb caused by pressure on a nerve at the wrist. Others report an inflammation of nerves in the arms, 'a pinching feeling all over the body', random muscular jerks, and a loss of the sense of smell. Researchers are studying more serious manifestations they have observed in patients to learn whether these are related to SS or to other underlying conditions. The investigators are also unsure of the causes of these conditions in SS. [47]

Lymphocytic Involvement

Sjogren's syndrome is a lympho-prolific condition; that is, the syndrome develops when the lymphocytes reproduce more freely than is normal in a non disease state. Those excess white cells infiltrate the tear glands, the saliva glands, and other glands or organs, interfering with their functioning and thus causing the dryness that is the hallmark of Sjogren's. It has been shown that these events often follow one another in stages. A person may first notice a swollen saliva gland and only years later develop a problem with dry eyes, etc. Most of the time these invasions are considered "benign". Although the presence of the extra cells does cause some damage, the immediate results are generally not serious. Long suffering victims may dispute having their problems being termed "not serious". I have always resented the television advertising that emphasizes the "minor aches of arthritis" when we all know that most of our aches are not minor at all! But all things are relative and in this case, 'serious' means life-threatening. The symptoms of SS are inconvenient and uncomfortable but for the most part do not affect the life span of the patients. However certain troublesome problems can arise. In some patients the unbridled multiplication of the lymphocytes tends to form clusters which doctors refer to as 'islands'. These groups of cells can give the appearance, in diagnostic tests, of tumors but may well not be malignant . In this case they are called 'pseudo lymphomas'. They must be carefully watched, since this 'imitation cancer' may develop into a real malignancy, a true lymphoma. This is one of the reasons your doctor will monitor your blood serum components regularly. A drop in the level of immunoglobulin where there was previously a high count, and a decrease in RA factor can signal an alert for the approaching lymphoma state and let the doctor know action needs to be taken. While it has been estimated that fewer than 5% of primary SS patients may develop lymphoma [63], as with all cancers, early diagnosis is extremely important. So your periodic blood checks take on added importance. Reassuring are the statistics that indicate an outcome of lymphoma is rare. In Sicca City, less than 25 of the primary SS patients can be concerned with the emergence of lymphoma. Dr. Talal does not want his patients to worry about that possibility. He tells them, "That's my job. I'm your doctor." He says, "I believe this. I don't take care of myself. I have a doctor. I let the doctor do the worrying for me." By way of reassurance, he says there are now sophisticated technologies to detect and diagnose lymphomas. They can be picked up at the earliest appearance and there is effective treatment. As for those few who do have lymphoma, at least half do not have it in the glands themselves so a swelling in the salivary glands usually doesn't mean lymphoma.

Symptoms 33

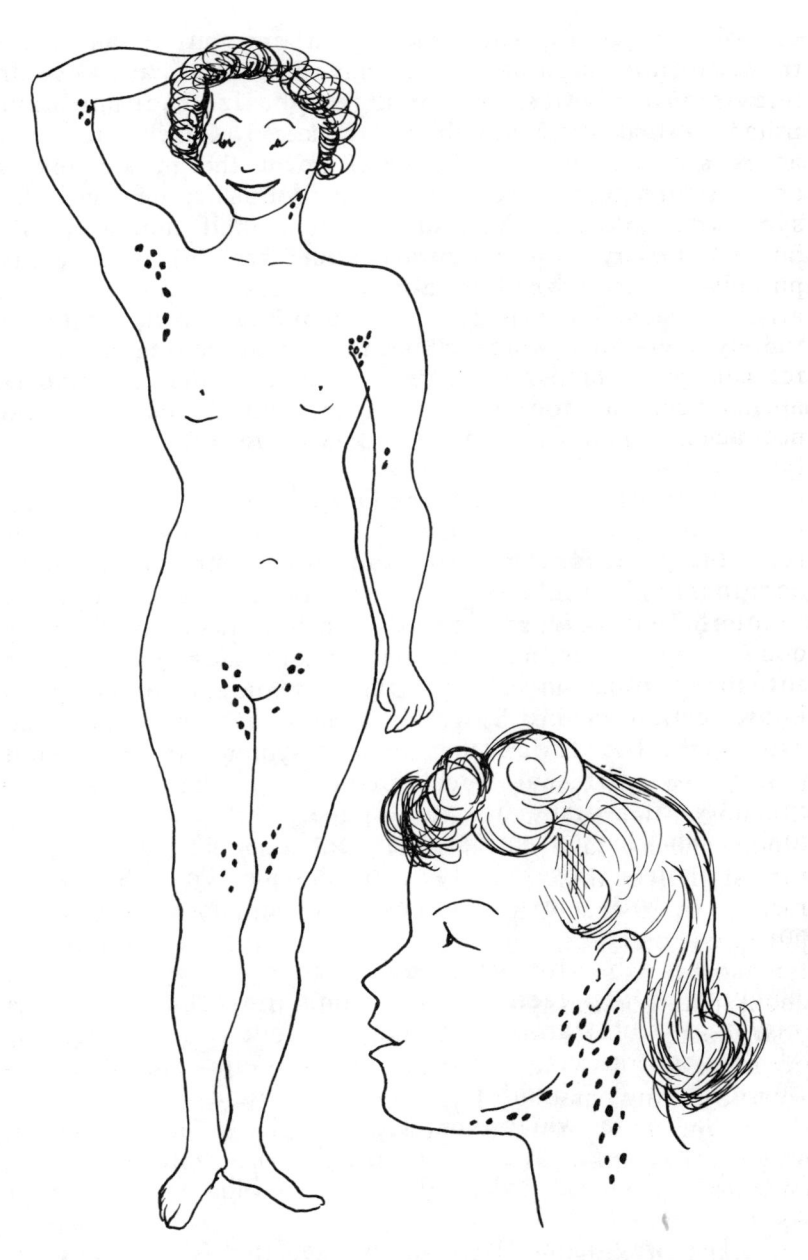

Figure 5 Lymph Nodes for Self-Examination

The patient can help by noting any changes in her condition such as swellings in the armpits or groin, or weight loss. He suggests a self examination similar to that done for breast cancer. Check the head and neck areas; behind the ears, down the neck muscle, and the armpits. An enlarged lymph node will be visible or palpable. You can see it, or if not, you can feel it. Why not examine your lymph node areas routinely along with the monthly breast exam?

But Dr. Talal insists you should not make a fetish of it. "You don't worry constantly about getting hit by a car, and you shouldn't worry about lymphoma. Patients should have a doctor they have confidence in, who understands Sjogren's and he'll take care of it."

Allergies

Many Sjogren's patients are troubled with allergies, particularly stuffy noses and rashes. Although a direct relationship has not been established, this is another area where diagnosis can be confusing, since many of the symptoms of allergic disease can also be Sjogren's symptoms. Actually, an allergic reaction is an immune system response but involves a different mechanism. That makes it especially important to distinguish the cause of the problem so that effective treatment can be carried out. If your stuffy nose really comes from your Sjogren's, treating it with anti-histamines can do more harm than good.

An allergic reaction happens when three elements are present: IgE, (immunoglobulin E), a proteinthat acts as an antibody, found in unusually high concentrations; white blood cells (mast cells) containing the chemical histamine; and an allergen the substance to which you are allergic. This could be almost anything: foods, feathers, the chemicals in detergents, pollens, even plain old mold or household dust.

The way it all happens is that the IgE latches on to a histamine-loaded mast cell. When this dynamic duo

Symptoms

sights the particles of pollen you have inhaled which are now circulating around your nasal passages, it lets fly with a blast of histamine. This irritating stuff brings on the itching, sneezing, and congestion we all know so well. This is a delayed reaction in that the first time you are exposed to a substance, you will not react but your immunoglobulins will be sensitized to it and remember. Sometime later, possibly the second time you are exposed, or possibly not till many years and many exposures later, the IgE/mast cell team will react unpleasantly when it recognizes that same allergen.

Of particular interest to the Sjogren's patient is the fact that these reactions could consist of a set of symptoms like a stuffed up head, post-nasal drip, congested ears, and swollen glands. Sound familiar? Right. All of these can also occur with SS and we are back to the old problem of mis-diagnosis. Maybe what you have treated as an allergy all these years is actually just one more aspect of your Sjogren's. But it is important to realize you can also have both. One does not necessarily exclude the other so both possibilities must be explored to determine the proper treatment.

Fatigue

A quick reading of the past chapter leaves one with little surprise at the information that Sjogren's syndrome generally brings fatigue and over-all weakness! Patients say they periodically feel drained of energy and need to rest during the day. One can be tooling along tending to business as usual and suddenly just 'crash'. Some patients must carefully conserve their energy but, fortunately for most of us, a short rest will usually restore the lost vim, at least for the time being.

Neonatal Lupus

Pregnant women who have, or suspect they may have Sjogren's syndrome should be aware of the possibility of a Lupus-like condition that can affect their baby. On exposure to sunlight, the baby may develop a rash much like that of a lupus patient. This is no cause for concern as it will go away of its own accord and does not need treatment. More serious is the heart blockage that can impair the infant's heart's ability to coordinate the beating of its valves, a possibly fatal defect. While some doctors have recommended abortion if a heart blockage is detected, current treatments can make that unnecessary. The heartblockage can now be overcome by the use of a pacemaker. While this only affects a small proportion of SS patients all mothers with Sjogren's antibodies (SS-A/antiRo) should be HLA typed early in their pregnancy and it is essential that they be carefully monitored with sonograms and other high risk pregnancy techniques. Be *sure* to tell your gynecologist (or any other doctor) about your Sjogren's syndrome! [80,5]

Secondary Sjogren's Syndrome

About 50 percent of all Sjogren's syndrome patients have the condition as a secondary manifestation of another connective tissue disease. It can be associated with rheumatoid arthritis, systemic lupus erythematosis, scleroderma, polymyositis, dermatomyositis or mixed connective tissue disease (MCTD) [2] Most frequently it co-exists with RA and, in fact, it has been hard, in the past, to tell if a patient actually has RA or just primary Sjogren's syndrome with strong symptoms mimicking RA. However, the criteria for separating the two conditions have been pretty well established in recent years.

Rheumatoid Arthritis

Rheumatoid arthritis is a systemic disease, afflicting many parts of the body. Symptoms may range from the minor discomfort of aching joints to crippling deformities of severe forms of the disease. Like Sjogren's syndrome, it is an auto-immune disease, in which certain antibodies in the bloodstream, turn against healthy cells instead of attacking invading disease cells. In RA the major targets are the joints. But it can also damage muscles, lungs, skin, blood vessels, nerves and eyes. These common symptoms bring about some of the confusion with Sjogren's syndrome, but there are tests to measure the blood factors that positively identify RA. As many as 25% of all RA patients also have Sjogren's syndrome.[14]

Systemic Lupus Erythematosus

An even higher percentage (up to 30%) of patients with SLE have Sjogren's syndrome, but, according to University of Texas Health Science Center immunologist Dr. Frank Arnett, distinguishing primary Sjogren's syndrome with lupus-like symptoms from Sjogren's syndrome secondary to lupus can still be a problem, even for the experts. When you consider that joint pain in hands, wrists, elbows, knees, or ankles; skin rashes; fatigue and weakness; and swollen glands are all early symptoms of lupus, you realize how a patient complaining of those things could be thought to have lupus when she may possibly have primary Sjogren's syndrome instead. Lupus, like Sjogren's syndrome, is a chronic, systemic, inflammatory auto-immune disease. Dr. Elaine Alexander, working at Johns Hopkins University, suggests that the close relationship of the two conditions may be the result of similar immunogenetic backgrounds of the patients. [5]

Like Sjogren's syndrome there are no cures but only ways to treat or to stave off problems. The lupus patient's skin will likely be extra sensitive to sunlight and he or she may experience a lack of appetite and muscle aches. Kidneys can be affected, and the linings of the heart and lungs could be attacked. The fact that depression often comes as a part of the illness is not surprising.[17]

Scleroderma

Four to five percent of all Sjogren's patients have associated scleroderma, again, a chronic, systemic, connective tissue disease   Once more the similarity is noted in the effects of the disease on the skin, joints, kidneys, blood vessels, digestive system, and the lungs. The muscles may also be attacked.   Raynaud's phenomenon (fingers sensitive to cold) is an early symptom of scleroderma.   Holding an icy cold drink glass in your hand, or getting angry triggers a narrowing of the small blood vessels of the fingertips causing the fingers to change color, first white and then blue, and tingle or turn numb.

Problems specific to scleroderma include swelling of the fingers or toes and a hardening of the skin from which the condition derives its name. "Sclero" comes from a Greek word meaning hardening; "derma" refers to skin.   Various internal organs and systems can be affected by this thickening process with an accompanying loss of function.[15]

Polymyositis and Dermatomyositis

In the myositis illnesses the immune system aims for the muscles, generating heat, redness, pain, and loss of function in those targets.   Since muscles provide the support of our bony framework, weakness is the end result of the inflammation of the muscles.   In dermatomyositis, skin rashes are evident along with the weakness.   The patient may develop purplish-red patches around the eyes   as Betty Rosen did.   Patients may have further symptoms such as fever, Raynaud's phenomenon, or, rarely, tumors.   Polymyositis and dermatomyositis are the least common of the diseases we are discussing with no more than 5 out of a million Americans being diagnosed each year.[13] Sicca City most likely doesn't have even one myositis patient. The statistic works out to one fourth of a patient for a city

Symptoms

of fifty thousand, but we wouldn't want to add to the poor person's troubles by chopping him up in quarters!

Conclusion

It's obvious by now that the symptoms of SS are far reaching and varied. Actually there are even more possible combinations of symptoms but they occur so rarely than it hardly seems worth adding them to an already too long list. Fortunately, no one patient is dealt a full hand of all these ills. In fact. that very difference from patient to patient adds to the complexity of the illness and produces an astonishingly diverse population of SS victims. It is helpful, too, to note once again, that there are many things doctor and patient can do to alleviate most of the listed symptoms. And even to prevent the more serious consequences of SS.

A suggestion that might be made here relates to being sure you remember to tell your doctor which of these symptoms you have noticed. No, you must not succumb to "medical student's disease." Just from reading about them you are likely to think you have every ache and pain mentioned. But wait a while. Set aside this book for a few days so your mind is not cluttered with all the "possibilities" mentioned in it. And then, why not draw your doctor a picture? Make a simple diagram of the human body (or photocopy the one in Figure 7) Now over a period of time, shortly before your next doctor's visit, just make marks wherever you have a problem. Use the spaces provided to make specific notes. For instance, "Eyes dry..need drops two or three times during night" or "Stiffness in the morning...goes away after I get up and move around." By making these notes as they occur to you, you won't be as likely to forget them when it's time to report to the doctor.

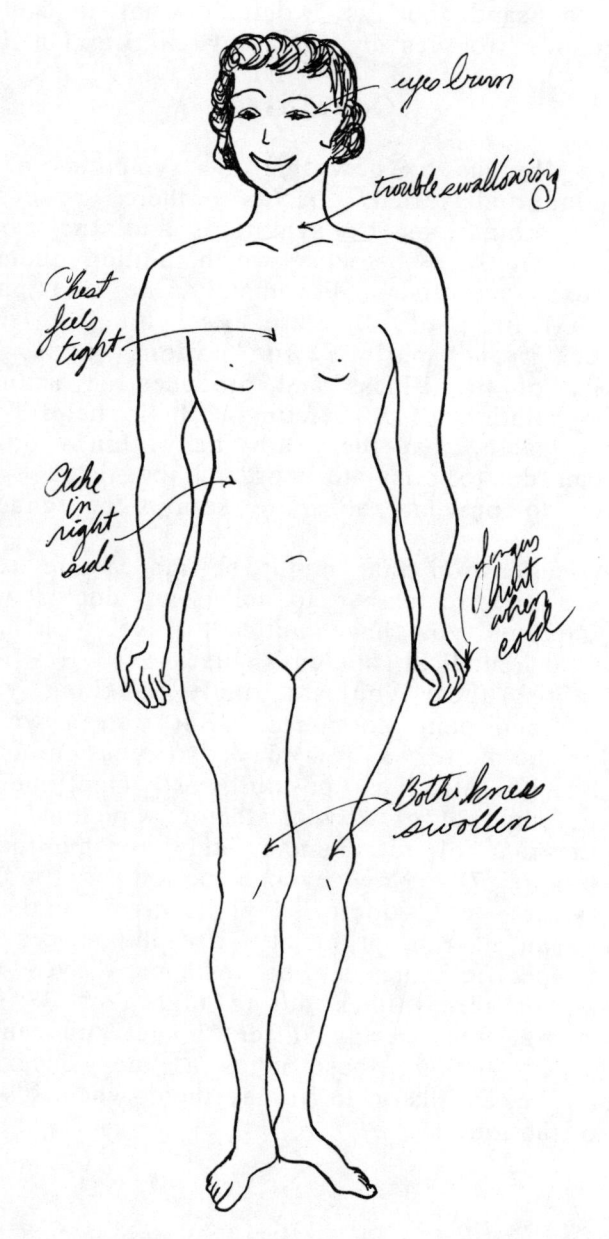

Figure 6   Figure Showing Complaints

Symptoms 41

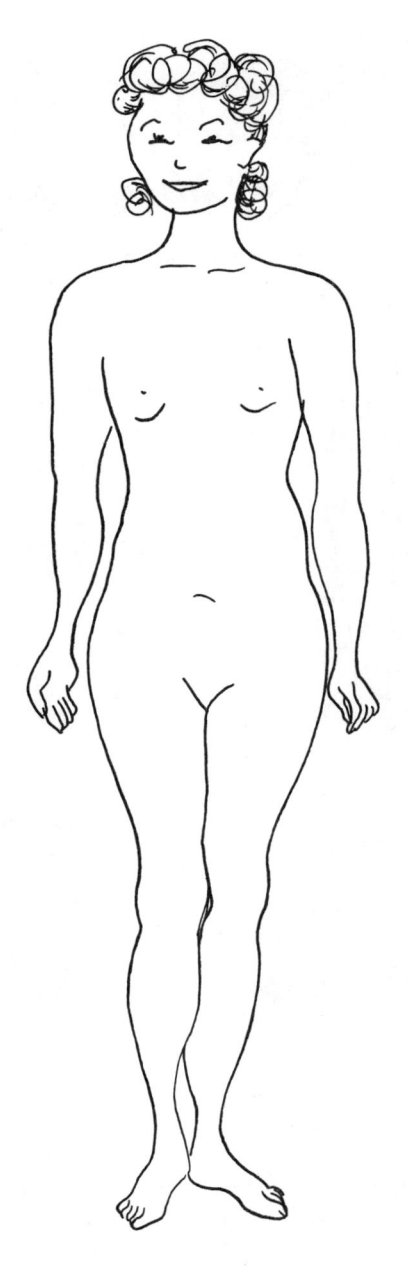

Figure 7 Figure Unmarked for Reader

Immunology

Chapter 3

What's Happening?

Since grade school days when Mrs. Murphy patiently tried to explain the intricacies of the human digestive system, I have been duly impressed. Our bodies are astonishingly complex machines. You have only to consider the structural design of the eye to be convinced of that. The old joke, "God must have known we'd eventually need to wear glasses; otherwise why would he put the ears where he did?" expresses my sense of wonder at the orderliness of our construction and the processes by which we operate.

The immune system is probably the most fascinating of all the departmentalized functions of the body. Even the most simplified description of the processes involved in protecting us from the forces bent on our destruction reads like a chronicle of global wars. A virtual army of white blood cells stands ready, at the first hint of foreign invasion, to mobilize itself against the threat. The troops consist of soldiers with names like phagocytes and lymphocytes, each with specific duties and skills to wage the battles. What's more, the various cells have a language by which they communicate strategies and the means to identify their enemies.

Only recently have scientists been able to begin to unravel the mysteries of how these things can be. Electron microscopes and revolutionary new technologies have allowed them to see and study and manipulate organisms so small the average person cannot even envision them. Tiny cells can now be magnified as much as 500,000 times and forced to reveal their secrets. So, though there are still many "holes" in the data, and new questions are constantly being raised, the researchers are beginning to be able to piece together the amazing drama that is constantly carried on within our bodies.

White Cell Warriors

Whenever an enemy agent, whether virus, bacteria, or protozoa, attacks us, it enters the body and seeks out the host cell it needs to reproduce and function. A virus, for instance, is not self-sufficient. It has only the instruction manual to carry out its work, not the necessary materials. For these it must locate and commandeer a particular type of cell. Using a specialized identification system, it locates the proper host, invades it and uses the cell's facilities to reproduce itself. These new viruses, in turn, break out of the cell to find new ones of their own to occupy, taking them over and repeating the process, creating many new viruses at each step. But all the while certain white blood cells that originate in the bone marrow, called phagocytes, have been cruising the body's blood vessel highways, keeping an eye out for trouble. When they spot it, they go into action quickly. Swift and efficient killers, they engulf the invading viruses and devour them. But the viruses can multiply faster than the phagocytes can consume them, so help

Immunology

is available from another group of white blood cells, the lymphocytes, or T cells. There are three types of T cells: the helpers, the killers and the suppressors. The first, the helpers, circulate constantly throughout the bloodstream, keeping the system under surveillance, like a scouting task force. When T cells programmed to recognize our particular unfriendly virus, spot the trouble the phagocytes are having, they come to the rescue. First they send out a call for reinforcements that brings more phagocytes and T cells to join the battle. But then they also go racing off to the nearest lymph node, where the back up troops, the killer T cells, are just waiting to be alerted. Stimulated by the helper cells, the killers hurriedly reproduce themselves, increasing their number substantially. These newly created soldiers then rush to the battle field. There they help out by killing off the infected host cells before the viruses can reproduce in them.

Meanwhile, back at the lymph node, the helper T cells have another job to do. They must also stir up yet another group of lymphocytes, the B cells. On orders from the helper cells, the B cells, like their T cell brothers before them, start to reproduce themselves. But at the same time, they begin to manufacture chemical weapons called antibodies (or immunoglobulins). The antibodies, specifically designed to attack the particular virus that's causing all the fuss, join the others at the battlefield and begin the work of destroying the viruses themselves, before the viruses can enter the host cells and begin to reproduce. Together with the phagocytes and killer T cells which have been holding the fort waiting for the slower B cells to do their work, the antibodies make short work of finishing off the invaders. From somewhere, no one is quite sure where, a contingent of "marines", non T cell types known as natural killer (NK) cells with the power to attack a variety of enemies, also joins the fray. 35 When the war is finally won, a new type of T cell, a suppressor cell, comes on the scene to sound the all clear, telling the killer cells and the B cells to take off for some R & R leave. The scavenging phagocytes, who, like goats, will eat anything, clean up the mess and the remaining T and B cells hang around, as memory cells, to make darn sure those bad guys don't come back. Or if they do, we're on the ready. It is this last feature that accounts for the immunity that develops after a person has once experienced a particular kind of disease, such as mumps.

Humoral Immunity

Two distinct types of action are going on in the warfare just described. The phagocytes, T cells, and B cells are engaged in a mechanical process using direct attacks on the cells to do their work. This is referred to as *cellular immunity*, while the action of the antibodies is chemical and since it takes place in the serum (a "humor", or functioning fluid) is known as *humoral immunity*. The antibodies, also known as immunoglobulins, are proteins specifically designed to combine with a certain antigen, the protein that identifies the invading virus. In doing so they serve several functions. They can hold down the virus so the phagocyte can more easily surround it; they can keep the virus from attaching to a host cell; or they can neutralize toxins put out by bacteria. Beyond this, these versatile warriors can simply blow up the enemy cell. There are many different kinds of antibodies which, in addition to targeting different enemy cells, belong to five separate classes programmed to serve different functions. Of particular interest to Sjogren's patients are those known as IgA. Secreted on mucous membranes they are capable of neutralizing viruses before they actually enter the body. One of the techniques of diagnosing Sjogren's involves the observation of excess concentrations of IgA in the saliva.

Immunology

System Breakdowns

Immune system diseases, and particularly auto immune disorders, are those that occur when some part of this elaborate protective system fails to function properly. From its very nature, one can see how there are many opportunities for malfunctions at various stages of the process. In some cases the invading virus can turn off the immune system, stopping the phagocytes and killer cells in their tracks. Sometimes the defenders become weakened by dietary lacks on the part of the host. Malnutrition cripples the thymus gland, the body's T cell producing factory. Some medications, particularly cancer chemotherapy can effectively suppress the immune system. In fact these same drugs are the ones used for that purpose in fighting the rejection of transplanted organs. Severe burns can seriously reduce the responsiveness of the immune system. But there is also a range of congenital defects that can result in immune deficiencies. And it is in this area that researchers think lies the basis for Sjogren's syndrome, as well as the other autoimmune diseases.

Autoimmunity

Probably the most amazing and puzzling aspect of the immune system is the ability of killer T cells and antibodies to recognize other cells, and to distinguish friend from foe. Each cell, and each invading entity (antigen) wears a badge, a genetic label constructed of proteins which, like a combination lock, are specific for one type of virus, hepatitis, for instance, and that one only. A killer cell programmed to intercept a hepatitis virus will completely ignore any other virus it bumps into on its journey, but immediately mobilize against any hepatitis virus it meets. The ability to know when NOT to react violently to another substance is called *immune tolerance* and it is the breakdown of immune tolerance that allows a confused T cell to attack the healthy tissues of its host.

A Trouble-making Trio

Researchers do not yet know what causes these self destructive attacks to occur, but they have recently concluded that, far from being a rare aberration that mysteriously appears in the bloodstream, the self destructive cells are there right along, but are being prevented from acting. Some studies show that helper T-cells somehow gain the upper hand over the suppressor T-cells whose job it is to keep them in check. It is the breakdown of these controls that is now thought to trigger the destructive course of RA, lupus, and the other autoimmune diseases, including Sjogren's syndrome. Still to be discovered are the factors that bring about the release of the dormant cells. Evidence points to a slow-growing virus, one that can hide, somehow, from the killer cells and live in the body many years in a cocoon-like state. Some event, a trauma or stressful situation, could activate the virus

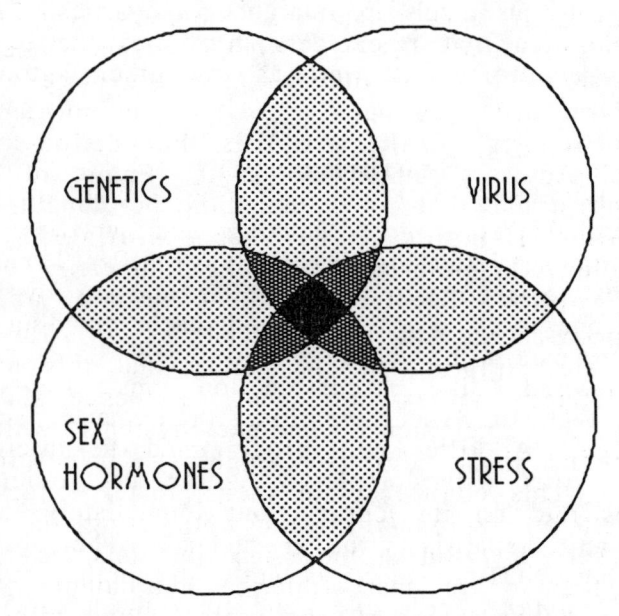

Figure 8 Factors in Autoimmunity
(Adapted from diagram by Dr. Norman Talal)

Immunology

and stimulate the T cells. So it becomes a possibility that the "cause" of Sjogren's is made up of three elements: an inherited genetic pre-disposition (self-destructive killer cells as part of the equipment some people are born with); a virus that gains entry early in life and lies in waiting; and an event that stirs both of them to action.

A person could have the genetic tendency to acquire an immune system disease, but never encounter the virus that would activate it. Or on the other hand, the virus would be rendered harmless if the mixed up T cells were not present or were never awakened. Under this theory, it would take the combination of all three circumstances to create a real live case of Sjogren's syndrome. [54]

Sexual Innuendos

A possible fourth element in the equation suggests itself in the fact that Sjogren's syndrome, and most autoimmune diseases, strike women much more often than men. Although this little piece of natural chauvinism had long been noted, it was not until 1972 that a report by the Arthritis Foundation-sponsored National Advisory Committee on the Future of Arthritis Research urged that an explanation be sought. Since that time, studies have been initiated at the Immunology laboratories at the University of Texas Health Science Center in San Antonio under Dr. Norman Talal and Dr. S. Ansar Ahmed. [74] Researchers there are exploring the possibility that this difference is moderated by sex hormones. Evidence shows that women have heightened immune systems which may strengthen their defenses against infections and tumors. This could explain their greater longevity and also help in reproduction, thus protecting the survival of the species. But at the same time this may be what makes them more susceptible to autoimmune diseases. On the other side of the coin, men with certain autoimmune diseases seem to have lower levels of male sex hormones. The ongoing studies are working to uncover exactly how the hormones act on the lymphocytes. [85]

Translating Causes to Effects

We have seen the sometimes devastating effects of the lack of moisture and discussed the possible reasons for the shortages but at times its hard to connect cause and effect. Why, for instance, would a simple loss of water in the mouth have all those repercussions? The answer lies in the fact that saliva is not simply 'water'. Far from it. It is a complex solution of ingredients with specific functions that are sorely missed by the SS patient.

Though predominantly water, saliva is also swimming with blood cells, immunoglobulins, enzyme containing proteins and lactoferrin, all carefully ph balanced. [67,43] All these components work together in the normal mouth to keep the natural balance in force. Antibodies gather together excess bacteria to be eliminated from the mouth. Enzymes deactivate them. Amino acids help control bacteria and fungus chloride thiocyanate, calcium, phosphate, and bicarbonate maintain the proper level of acidity and alkalinity while the calcium and phosphates in the saliva stand ready to replenish any lack of those minerals on the teeth. Lactoferrin (a natural saliva component) in normal amounts helps protect the mouth from bacterial infections, but in the increased quantities found in SS, upsets the normal migration patterns of the T cells, attracting them like a magnet to the affected glands, and actually contributing to the tissue destruction. [39] I'll bet you won't ever again think of saliva as just mouth water! The saliva glands bring to mind a chocolate factory in which various ingredients are poured from assorted tubes into enormous vats and constantly blended to make just the right mix. Hold back some of the sugar and the gooey stuff is too bitter. Too much of another ingredient and it might not be the

Immunology

right consistency. In saliva the composition is regulated by the glands' activity. The flow rate changes as needed and is influenced by many factors such as your diet. Thus sweet treats stimulate it and certain foods, persimmons, for instance, can dry it up in a hurry. Thus the famous pucker. But it is not just the amount but the actual proportion of ingredients that changes. Not only that but the glands can get tired from all that busywork. After that great Christmas dinner, they definitely need a rest and time to refill their tanks. SS patients learn to be extremely careful what they put in their mouths, and when.

Why me?

It is almost impossible not to wonder, specifically, where do I come in? How did I get involved in all this? And should my children be worried about getting it? What about their children? When a young prospective parent asks me that question, my best answer is that none of my problems has yet made me wish I hadn't been born. But it is of legitimate concern to patients and their families. And to the doctors trying to solve the puzzles.

In most cases, a person who has Sjogren's syndrome has never heard of it before diagnosis. No one she knows and no one in her family has it. Studies to determine if Sjogren's syndrome is inherited, and indicate that certain genetic factors that show up in the blood of the majority of patients. These factors have been identified as anti-Ro (SS-A) and anti-La(SS-B) antibodies, and HLA-DR2, DR3 and DRw52 antigens. Immunologists are still studying the patterns of occurrence of these factors and their implications for the likelihood of a particular person getting Sjogren's syndrome. More, they are hopeful that this information will help predict the probable course of the disease. Thus, if it is found that a patient has a certain component of genes, this person will be more or less likely to have serious complications, which in turn, can then be anticipated and treated as required.

Also, some components have been found to cross the boundaries of the various diseases. Part of the difficulty in diagnosing SS lies in the fact that it shares some blood factors with rheumatoid arthritis, and even more so with lupus. Seeing an indicator of lupus (or RA) in the blood chemistry can lead to a confused impression that lupus (or RA) is present.

In studies of families, a cluster of different autoimmune diseases is more often found than a grouping of several members with the same disease. An SS patient's sister may have RA, while a cousin has scleroderma, but it is rare for several members of the same family all to have SS. The author's mother had a swollen parotid gland removed as a child (That was around the turn of the century and she is now, at 92, well and chipper with no sign of autoimmune illness!). Her brother had multiple sclerosis (thought to have an autoimmune origin) [6], and an aunt had a thyroid disease (goiter). Since it has also been shown that affected family members do not necessarily share the same HLA complexes [64], it is believed that a combination of genetic effects (hereditary predisposition) and environmental triggers influence the disease statistics. Identifying these elements may even lead eventually to ways to prevent the development of immune disorders[12]

Important to this hope is the ability to distinguish between primary and secondary SS. As we have stated, sicca syndrome is considered primary when it occurs without any other well-defined rheumatic disease. When the rheumatic disease is present, the Sjogren's is considered secondary. The patient suffering from acutely dry eyes and mouth may not be much concerned at the moment with being put in a particular pigeonhole. Both sets of victims are likely to have these problems, and aching joints, too. After all, that is the definition we have already set up. Two out of three symptoms lets you into the not so exclusive club of Sjogren's syndrome. But there are significant differences. Obviously, its a relief if you

Immunology

hear, as I did, "there's no way you could have had RA for twenty years and show no sign of it in the joints of your hands." Those words lifted the sentence I had been under for all those years; the specter of an old age marred by crippling deformities and possibly spent in a wheelchair. On the other side of the coin, if you do have RA, the effects of the Sjogren's are likely to be less disturbing. But more importantly, the distinctions still being revealed by ongoing research will make the management of the condition much more accurate. Studies indicate that instead of a catchall situation, we are dealing with two distinct entities. The differences are clearly indicated not only in clinical manifestations but also in the serologic and genetic markers. Where the circulating antibodies mentioned earlier are positive signs of Sjogren's syndrome, some are predominantly present in PSS and absent in RA-SS and some just the opposite. Both situations may carry the RA factor and antinuclear antibodies (indicative of lupus) even though the primary SS patient does not actually have those diseases. Both can also show the SS-A and SS-B antibodies in about equal proportions, but the presence of SS-A seems to indicate a greater possibility of complications such as vasculitis. Antibodies against salivary ducts appear much more frequently in secondary SS. The antigens HLA-B8 [58] and HLA-DR3 are associated most often with primary SS, while HLA-Dw52 (MT2)[36] is found in both.

Symptoms that help differentiate include more frequent swelling of the face, jaws, or neck; and more of a need to make those night time trips to the bathroom. Thyroid involvement, showing up as sluggishness, is most often seen in primary SS. The primary form also more commonly includes the smarting fingers (Raynaud's phenomenon), the burgundy colored skin splotches (purpura), and muscle weakness (myositis).[58] The joint painsof primary SS are generally milder and most often affect the smaller joints, without, as we have noted, bringing on the deformity of those joints.

Chapter 4

History

The story of our knowledge of Sjogren's syndrome is one of many doctors picking up on the different symptoms in different patients and gradually piecing together the picture of the systemic disease described in this book. It is a process that covered the work of a good number of doctors over a period of years.

Filamentary Keratitis

The story begins on a particular day in 1882, when the Eye Clinic at Heidelberg Congress was holding an afternoon session.[70] Dr. Leber reported on three patients who particularly interested him. In each of the three, he had noticed strands or filaments attached to the corneas of the eyes. The strands were removed, but grew back. Leber called the condition filamentary keratitis. The next year Dr. Uhtoff showed drawings he had made of similar filaments which some viewers declared to look like coiled snakes or perhaps a garden hose.

Swollen Glands

When 42-year-old Christof Kalweit left his farm near Vienna to seek the help of the young doctor Johann von Mikulicz-Radecki, he was worried about puffy swellings around his eyes that were interfering with his sight. The enlarged tear glands were later echoed by swollen saliva glands. Mikulicz, surgical assistant to famed surgeon Dr. Christian Albert Theodore Billruth, removed the tumors but they reappeared two months later. There was a second operation and by the time Kalweit died of appendicitis several months later, the swellings were almost gone.
Wishing to honor his mentor, Dr. Billruth, Mikulicz gave a paper describing the case before a symposium honoring the professor's academic achievements. And again in 1892, as a professor himself at Breslau, he published an account of Kalweit's history, noting that the condition was mild but with a tendency to relapse. Unfortunately, Mikulicz' work led to a confusing lumping of a variety of salivary gland conditions under his name, in spite of the fact that the doctor had clearly detailed the atrophy brought on by cell infiltrations of the glands in his patients. There was much confusion among medical circles as doctors rushed to get on the bandwagon, describing every case of swollen glands they saw as Mikulicz' disease. In 1907, a Dr. Napp proclaimed it to be merely a collection of symptoms that could be brought on by any number of other causes. By 1914 Dr. Thursfield had divided the syndrome into eight separate categories which were regrouped in 1927 back down to two groups classified as Mikulicz' disease resulting from known causes or Mikulicz' disease resulting from unknown causes.

History

Xerostomia

In the meantime the association of dry eyes and a dry mouth, which he christened "xerostomia", was reported by Dr. W. B. Hadden in 1888, but it took Dr. Fuchs, writing in 1919, to make the connection between tear gland deficiency and dry eyes as well as the association of swollen salivary glands and dryness of the mouth.

Gougerot's syndrome

In the early twenties, the French physician, Dr. H. Gougerot maintained that a general condition existed in which the eyes, mouth, larnyx, nose, and vulva all suffered from a related dryness which also affected the thyroid and ovaries. In fact, the syndrome is still referred to in France as "Gougerot's syndrome".

Arthritis

An elderly patient crippled with arthritis and at the same time, suffering from the same filamentary cornea disease (keratitis) attracted the attention of Mulock Houwer in 1927. He began noticing that other patients had the same combination of symptoms, adding the third element of the syndrome, a finding confirmed by other studies and other physicians.

Sjogren's Keratoconjunctivitis

Swedish ophthalmologist Henrik Sjogren, fascinated by his first case of dry eyes, began a careful study of the condition in 1930. Born in October, 1899, in the Swedish town of Koping, young Henrik completed his medical studies at Stockholm's Karolinska Institute in 1927. He met Maria Hellgren, the daughter of a prominent ophthalmologist, composed a delightful waltz to honor their engagement, and married her while still in training for his own ophthalmology specialty at Serafimerlasarettet in Stockholm. During that time Sjogren saw a particular patient who piqued his interest. At 49, the woman had no tears for crying and couldn't swallow her food without a drink to wash it down. She had come in complaining of the 'rheumatismus chronicus' that had bothered her for six years and the burning, itching sensation of a foreign body in her eyes. Intrigued, he checked her eyes with rose-bengal staining and observed dry spots on her corneas.

After seeing four other similar cases the same year, Sjogren wrote them up for the Swedish Medical Association journal _Hygiea._ In that comprehensive report published in 1933, he dubbed the condition "keratoconjunctivitis sicca" He concluded that keratoconjunctivitis was only part of a larger complex of symptoms which involved the tear glands, the saliva glands, the mucous glands of the nasal passages, and swollen jaws. He noted the frequency of arthritis as an additional symptom.

Unfortunately for Sjogren, his thesis *Zur Kenntnis der Keratoconjunctivitis Sicca'*, was not as highly praised then as it is now and he was denied the necessary rank as Docent. As a result, he didn't pursue an academic career. Instead he joined the staff of a hospital in southern Sweden where he continued his research. Sjogren was responsible for the adoption of the Schirmer test and rose bengal staining as diagnostic tools. (See Chapter 4, Diagnosis and Testing). Sjogren's 20 years of work in identifying and recording the parameters of the disease was first honored with his name in 1936 when Von Grosz applied the name "Sjogren's syndrome" to the sicca complex. By the early forties his name was firmly attached to the syndrome he described and his once unappreciated thesis was translated into English and widely circulated.

He continued publishing papers and giving talks on SS, making his way around the world and receiving many honors from the medical world. In 1957 he was finally awarded the title of Docent from the University of Gothenburg. He has been named to honorary

History

membership in the American Rheumatism Association, the Swedish Rheumatology Society, and the Royal College of Physicians and Surgeons of Glasgow.[91]

At the time of the Copenhagen Symposium, he was living at the Ribbingska home in Lund, Sweden, still alert and keeping up with scientific literature. Death claimed him on the 17th of September, 1986.[50]

Sjogren's vs Mikulicz

Other researchers followed, discovering the frequent association of Sjogren's syndrome with rheumatoid arthritis. Dr. S. Holm noted the similarities, but it was not until 1953 that the team of Dr. Winfield Morgan and Dr. Benjamin Castleman, presented a paper [57] before the Boston gathering of the New England Pathological Society n 1950 and the Fiftieth Annual meeting of the American Association of Pathologists and Bacteriologists in St. Louis in 1953, concluding that Sjogren and Mikulicz were actually describing the same disease. Sjogren himself had written that they should be thought of separately, even publishing a table to illustrate his reasoning. Morgan and Castleman started out studying Mikulicz' disease to discover what made the parotid glandact as it did in that syndrome. They recorded the findings that showed the lymphocytes replaced the gland's secreting cells, the multiplication of mucus secreting cells and the clumping of connective tissue cells.[70]. Later, while reviewing the cases of that study, Morgan found a significant number of cases where the patients had the three parts of Sjogren's syndrome: the dry eyes, the dry mouth, and the arthritis Not only that, but an analysis of one of Sjogren's patients revealed changes just like the ones Morgan and Castleman had described, and in fact they were just as Mikulicz had seen them, sixty-five years earlier. The two syndromes were actually one. Even in those days the confusion came about because no two patients were exactly alike. As Shearn wrote in 1971, "Those patients with dry eyes saw an ophthalmologist, whereas those with salivary gland involvement were seen by a surgeon or otolaryngologist. In a similar fashion, the internist and rheumatologist studying the articular manifestations of a patient might be totally unaware of the seemingly unimportant complaints of dry eyes or recurring parotitis."

Ongoing Research

In the years since Morgan and Castleman's original study, much has been done to further refine the criteria for diagnosis of Sjogren's. The American Rheumatism Association standards demonstrated the "intimate relationship" of Sjogren's syndrome with rheumatoid arthritis, scleroderma, polymyositis polyarteritis, systemic lupus erythematosis, purpura hyperglobulinemia (a blood condition), and Hashimoto's thyroiditis (an inflammation of the thyroid gland). Dr. Hashimoto himself recognized the similar changes of the thyroid glands he studied and the salivary glands Mikulicz reported on. Continuing studies expand our knowledge of the diversity of Sjogren's syndrome. We'll explore later the work of researchers across the country that is ongoing in the 80s. The studies not only deal with the ramifications of the disease but also look into the probable hereditary and triggering factors that bring about the changes of Sjogren's syndrome.

Chapter 5

Diagnosis and Testing

All right, if you've read this far, you surely have dry eyes and aches and pains all over your body. It could be what's known as "Medical Student's Disease". The power of suggestion. Every student in every medical school suffers from all the symptoms he studies about. But if you've have had for a long time, some of the symptoms you've read about here, it's probably making you wonder. How can the average person know if those symptoms mean he (or she) has Sjogren's syndrome? It's worth mentioning them to your doctor. He or she can investigate the possible causes. For every symptom that can be part of SS, there are assorted other possible causes. Dry eyes can be the result of chemicals in the air, dust irritation, or certain medications. Drugs can also dry up your mouth and throat, as can cigaret smoking or chemotherapy. We all know many things can make the joints ache. The biggest villain of all can be simple stress. The deadline you have to meet at the office or the husband who drives you up the wall can put a crick in your neck faster than a chilling draft. A rugged tennis game can wreck your elbows and Grandma insists it's the rain comin' tomorrow that does it. But if those problems go away and the aches don't, its time to see your doctor and tell all. He can use many tests and diagnostic procedures to pin down the source of the trouble.

The Copenhagen Symposium and the Four Criteria

As has been indicated before, one of the most frustrating things about SS is the problem of diagnosis. Three or four medical organizations who have set up criteria for establishing a clinical diagnosis of SS, but none agree totally. In September, 1986, the First International Symposium on Sjogren's Syndrome was held in Copenhagen, Denmark under the leadership of Dr. Jan Prause of the University of Copenhagen Institute of Eye Pathology, and Dr. Rolf Manthorpe of Sweden's University of Lund Papers were presented by doctors from the US, Denmark, Sweden, Canada, England, Greece, Japan, and other countries.

One of the main items of business was to establish an international set of criteria for the diagnosis of Sjogren's syndrome. This is extremely important, not only for the identification of patients but for the orderly progress of the research being done around the world. Standards must be formed and maintained in order for one set of studies, in Japan, for instance, to be relevant in respect to another set being carried out in Greece. Four different organizations came to the conference with their own sets of rules, referred to as the Copenhagen, the Japanese, the Greek, and the California criteria. Each was discussed separately and comparatively assessed with the goal of choosing the factors needed to make a single code to be used by all doctors and researchers. Dr. Manthorpe headed a

Diagnosis/Testing

committee presenting comments on the four criteria.48

It was basic that the syndrome involved, by definition, the eyes, the mouth and the joints. But research has shown that the disease is an autoimmune disorder encompassing many different organs of the body as well as the exocrine glands. All parts of the body dependent on lubricating secretions for proper functioning must be considered in the overall picture of Sjogren's syndrome. To evaluate these involvements, it was noted that several tests should be made for each organ, the number depending on how specific the available tests are. If a test had been devised that will give a particular result ONLY if Sjogren's is present it alone would be sufficient. But at this date, most tests can give positive results from other causes. We have seen that allergy medications, among others, can cause both dry eyes and dry mouth. But if a patient tells the doctor she feels the dryness (subjective evidence), a scintigram shows decreased secretion, and a lip biopsy confirms the presence of lymphocytes, it points specifically to SS as the cause of the oral dryness. It is essential that all the study centers use the same methods of testing.

Similarly, the terminology must be standard. Much of the history of confusion about SS arises from the use of different terms with vague meanings. Dry eye has been called 'xerosis' or 'xerophthalmia', but the latter word is firmly identified with a lack of vitamin A and the term now generally accepted is Henrik Sjogren's own cumbersome, but certainly specific, keratoconjuntivitis sicca. That one is easy to recognise in writing but just wait until you hear an experienced doctor rattle it off rapidly!

A third problem is the distinction between objective and subjective abnormalities. Not only do some patients report dryness when there is no definite indication in the tests, but other patients may have positive test factors without complaining of noticeable symptoms. Perhaps it has been so long since their eyes felt 'normal', they no longer remember what it was like. In Copenhagen, the doctors insist that only the abnormalities that can be measured accurately should be considered. In California, they use mostly the strict tests, but also look for 'symptoms' of dry mouth, etc. In Japan and Greece, the patients must have complaints about the dry eyes and mouth in addition to the positive test scores. Blood tests and biopsies also carry different importance to the different investigators. The Japanese, Greek, and Californian criteria distinguish between a 'definite' and 'probable' diagnosis, while only the Copenhagen and the Greek groups separate primary from secondary SS, a situation the reviewers disagreed with. The symposium report concluded that in addition to observing a unified criteria, the tests used and their normal ranges should be noted in any reports of studies published in future scientific journals. That way all of the knowledge being painstakingly accumulated will increase the total information.

The Criteria Compared

The Copenhagen Criteria: Primary Sjogren's syndrome occurs if patient has keratoconjunctivitis or KCS (dry eyes) *and* xerostomia (dry mouth) but does not meet international criteria for another chronic inflammatory connective tissue disease. KCS and xerostomia each require abnormal test results from two of the three following tests. For KCS: 1. The Schirmer-I test, 2. The break-up time (BUT), 3. The van Bijsterveld score (rose-bengal staining). For xerostomia: 1. Unstimulated sialogram, 2. Salivary gland scintigram, 3. Lower lip biopsy. [48]

The Greek Criteria: Definite primary SS equals two out of three of the following: For xerophthalmia: Patient complains of eyes feeling dry, Schirmer's test abnormal, or positive rose-bengal staining. For xerostomia: patient complains of dry mouth, parotid flow rate is low, and the parotid glands are or have been swollen. All patients must have biopsy showing excess lymphocytes. [72]

Diagnosis/Testing

The Japanese Criteria: All patients must have symptoms of dry mouth and eyes plus positive rose-bengal and Schirmer's tests along with abnormal findings on lip biopsy and sialogram. [34]

The California Criteria: 1 For KCS, Schirmer's test must show decreased tear flow and there must be increased staining with rose-bengal or fluorescein dye. For xerostomia, dry symptoms must be backed up by decreased salivary flow rates. A biopsy must show excessive lymphocytes and there must be laboratory evidence of a systemic autoimmune disease. [28]

The overlapping and confusing elements of these criteria sets are graphically shown on Figure 9. Since the criteria generally do agree on the presence of dry eyes and dry mouth as important to the diagnosis, these are the first areas that will be tested once a patient has confessed to not liking saltines and having eye problems. But even the various tests now in use can be problematical. J. M. Gumpel put it well in his comments in the British Medical Journal.[30] "The results of diagnostic tests for Sjogren's syndrome," he says," tend to be positive when the diagnosis is obvious, and equivocal when one most needs them."

Dry Eyes - Keratoconjunctivitis

For the eyes, two major tests will be administered by your ophthalmologist. First, the Schirmer Test consists of placing short strips of filter paper inside the lower eyelid. This, as you might imagine, smarts, as it is intended to. We are supposed to, literally, have a bawl. The measurement depends on the amount of tears produced and the resulting wetness of the filter paper. A length of wetness of less than 5 millimeters is considered abnormal and an indication of SS.

A more accurate test is the rose bengal staining method in which dye is placed in the eye and it is examined thru a slit lamp. That's that devilishly bright light the doctor shines in your eyes so he can see what's going on. The stain takes better on damaged

SJOGREN'S DIAGNOSTIC CRITERIA

KERATOCONJUNCTIVITIS SICCA (KCS)

   SCHIRMER TEST

   Wet ≤ 10 mm / 5 Min.
   Wet < 10 mm / 5 Min.
   Wet < 9 mm / 5 Min.
   Wet ≤ 5 mm / 5 Min.

   ROSE-BENGAL STAINING

   van Bijsterveld score > 4, out of 9
   Positive staining (++ or more)
   Positive staining

   BREAK-UP TIME (BUT) ≤ 10 Sec.
   FLUORESCEIN TEST   (Positive)

XEROSTOMIA

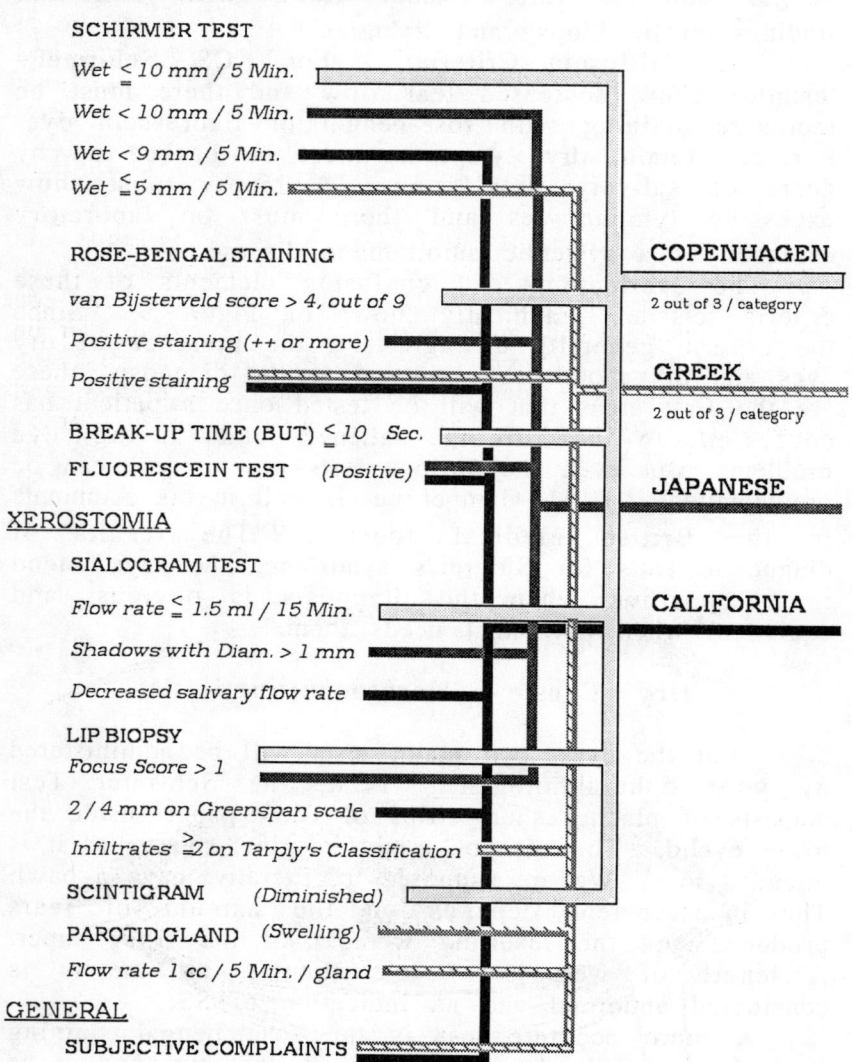

   SIALOGRAM TEST

   Flow rate ≤ 1.5 ml / 15 Min.
   Shadows with Diam. > 1 mm
   Decreased salivary flow rate

   LIP BIOPSY

   Focus Score > 1
   2 / 4 mm on Greenspan scale
   Infiltrates ≥ 2 on Tarply's Classification

   SCINTIGRAM   (Diminished)
   PAROTID GLAND   (Swelling)
   Flow rate 1 cc / 5 Min. / gland

GENERAL

   SUBJECTIVE COMPLAINTS

COPENHAGEN
2 out of 3 / category

GREEK
2 out of 3 / category

JAPANESE

CALIFORNIA

Figure 9   Sjogren's Syndrome Diagnostic Criteria Compared

Diagnosis/Testing

surfaces so the amount of staining he sees tells him the degree of dryness.

Still another test measures the length of time the tear film lasts between blinks. Normally it should be at least 15 seconds before the film begins to breakup and dry spots appear. This breakup time (BUT) is also checked during a slit lamp examination.

Dry mouth - Xerostomia

The involvement of the salivary glands is determined by a combination of observation and tests. Swellings of the glands along the cheekline can be more or less obvious and the inside of the mouth can be seen to be dry. Nuclear scanning measures the function of all the major salivary glands accurately and painlessly. Injections of dye can also be useful for x-raying the parotid glands.

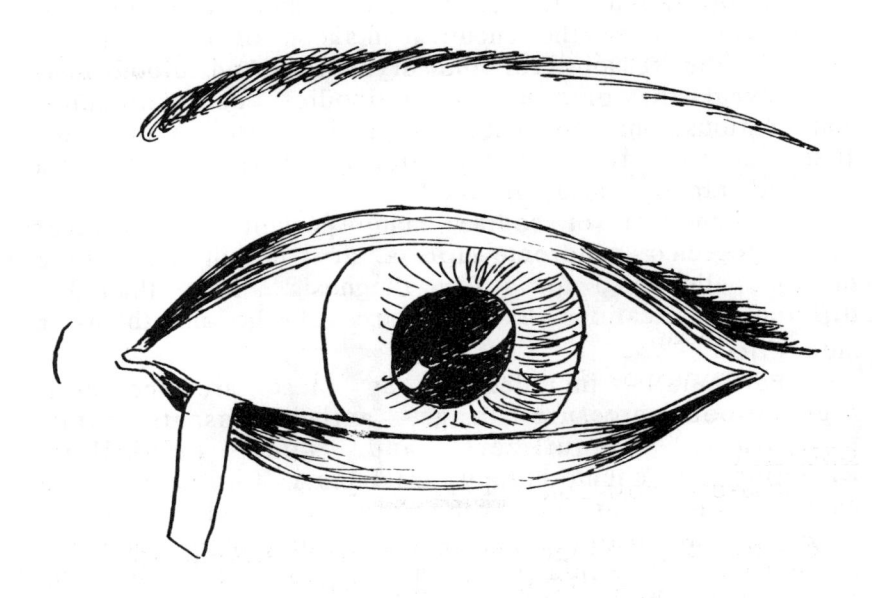

Figure 10 Schirmer Test

Scinti-scans use isotopes to identify a malfunctioning gland. The most effective confirmation of an oral Sjogren's syndrome diagnosis comes from a tissue sample (biopsy) of the saliva glands found on the inside of the lower lip. This can be examined under a microscope where the infiltrating lymphocytes can be counted. [10] When 50 or more inflammatory cells are found in a 4 millimeter square section of glandular tissue, the tissue is said to have a focus score of one, Anything greater than one is considered abnormal. and an indication of SS. [69] The researchers at the National Institute of Dental Research have developed still better methods of testing the salivary glands They can now measure the flow of saliva from glands that have been stimulated by chewing or sucking on sour candies, etc. and comparing that with the flow when glands have not been stimulated, such as when sleeping or resting. A contraption called a periotron measures the electrical resistance of tiny amounts of saliva collected on a small piece of filter paper, providing a digital readout of the amount of saliva put out by one gland in 2 minutes. They also analyze the chemical makeup of the saliva to discover the reasons for the dryness. And blood tests can reveal the presence of antibodies, auto-antibodies, and various markers that point to SS. All too often the first clue we have is the painful messages we get from our too rapidly decaying teeth.

There are, of course, many possible causes other than Sjogren's syndrome for a dry mouth and these must be eliminated for a firm diagnosis. More than 300 different medications have dryness of the mouth as a side effect. [59]

Particularly included among these are the anti-high blood pressure drugs, anti-depressants, anti-histamines, tranquilizers and some painkillers. Radiation or chemotherapy treatments for cancer can cause dryness, as can other diseases and conditions such as nutritional deficiencies and bone marrow transplants. It would be a mistake to assume any one cause for the problem without proper diagnostic

Diagnosis/Testing

testing, though it has been all too commonly done in the past. It is also important to mention here that the tests are not infallible and should be repeated for a follow-up. A negative Schirmer test or lip biopsy can be followed later by a positive test and many factors must be taken into consideration.

Unisom	Elavil	Aldoril
RuTus	Parsidol	Dristan
Donatol	Tofranil	Marijuana
Dimetane	Polaramine	Morphine
Caladryl	Triaminic	Benadryl
Primatine	Nitrous Oxide	Actifed
4 Way Nasal Spray		Inderal
Maximum Strength Midol		

Figure 11 Medications That May Cause Dry Eyes or Mouth

Arthritis

Examination for the relatively mild joint pains that accompany primary SS may be mostly subjective. That is the patient telling the doctor the extent of his or her aches and pains. But the doctor will want to pursue this by ordering blood tests to check for the presence of rheumatoid factors or anti-nuclear antibodies. These are the indicators for rheumatoid arthritis and lupus, respectively, and are frequently present in numbers too small to count as having the disease. The antibodies known as SS-A and SS-B are signals for a diagnosis of Sjogren's syndrome.

Extraglandular

Other tests to check for involvement of specific organs may be needed. These may include, for example, urine tests for kidney function, chest xrays to examine lungs, or thyroid function tests. A relatively new technique, magnetic resonance imaging is an extremely sensitive procedure for detecting signs of nervous system involvement and distinguishing SS/CNS from the diseases it tends to mimic; multiple sclerosis, Alzheimers and Parkinsons.[80] This is important, since, according to Dr. Alexander, unlike those other cases, the memory problems of SS are potentially treatable if diagnosed early.

Secondary Sjogren's Syndrome

However, as we have noted before, about fifty percent of all SS patients have some form of connective tissue disease along with their SS; so it is important to establish the presence or absence of another disease. Generally, it has been observed that in secondary SS, the other disease is noticed and diagnosed first, but a patient should always be observed for any changes that develop during treatment.

Rheumatoid Arthritis

The most common associated disease is rheumatoid arthritis and since it, like SS, affects the body many ways, it can take a combination of methods and possibly a fair amount of time to arrive at a firm diagnosis. The doctor will study your affected joints for signs of swelling, inflammation or distortion. In addition to checking your blood for RA factor, he may order a sed rate (erythrocyte sedimentation rate) test which measures the speed with which the red blood cells sink to the bottom of a test tube. RA patients have a faster rate of fall than others. During this same lab workup, your blood will probably be checked for red cell count

Diagnosis/Testing

or anemia. There may be other tests made from blood or urine and though x-rays tend not to show any abnormalities at the beginning, they may be taken to serve as a measure for changes later.

Lupus

The second most common associated disease is lupus (systemic lupus erythematosis or SLE. This one is even more complicated than RA to diagnose. Similar blood tests will be done, this time looking for the ANA(anti-nuclear antibody) proteins that are a marker for lupus. Essentially the same tests as for RA will be done plus, possibly, chest x-rays and an electrocardiogram. If the doctor thinks the kidneys may be involved, he may order a biopsy of that organ.

Scleroderma

A few SS patients (4 to 5% estimated, 40 to 50 Sicca Citians) also have scleroderma. Tests specifically designed to establish the presence of scleroderma may include a skin biopsy and a check of the muscle pressure of your esophagus to measure digestive system involvement, if any. Blood work is needed here also, and since scleroderma is complicated, some patients may be asked to enter the hospital for a short stay for more diagnostic tests.

Chapter 6

Treatment

By this time you may be wondering, what's the point? Arthritis is chronic and incurable, right? So's this Sjogren's syndrome thing. So why go to all this bother to figure out what you've got or which one you've got? Reading about all these symptoms just makes it worse and all those tests are an expensive nuisance. Maybe we'd all be better off not knowing. I hate needles anyway.

True, there is, at this point, no cure for Sjogren's syndrome. Or any of the related connective tissue diseases. But there are ways to treat the symptoms and prevent or alleviate the consequences.

The care program that you and your doctor will work out can be broken down into three areas. A combination of medication, careful observation and exercise, specifically tailored for your needs, will help you feel better and make life easier for you.

Dry Eyes

The most important thing for your eyes is to protect them from irritation by replacing the moisture the tear glands can no longer supply. For this we use artificial tears. There is an assortment of non-prescription artificial tears available at your local drug store. Some are methylcellulose based and some use

Major Ingredient	Trade Name	Preservatives	Benzalkonium chloride	Chlorobutanol	Edate disodium	Methylparaben	Propylparaben	Thimersal	None
Hydroxy Propyl Cellulose	Lacrisert								◊
Hydroxy Propyl Methyl Cellulose	Lacril		◊	◊					
	Tearisol			◊					
Polyvinyl Alcohol	Liquifilm Tears			◊					
	Liquifilm Forte				◊			◊	
	Tears Plus			◊					
Hydroxy Ethyl Cellulose	Clerz				◊			◊	
	Lyteers		◊		◊				
Methyl Cellulose	Methopto		◊						
	Methulose		◊						
	Murocel					◊	◊		
Other Polymeric Systems	Adaptettes		◊	◊				◊	
	Adsorbotar			◊				◊	
	Comfort Drops		◊	◊					
	Hypotears			◊					
	Tears Naturale		◊◊	◊					
Polyvinyl Alcohol + Cellulose Ester	Contique WS		◊◊						
	Lensine 5								
	Liquifilm WS		◊◊						
	Neo-Tears								
	Visalene WS		◊					◊	
Gum Cellulose	Gum Cellulose								◊

Figure 12 Artificial Tear Ingredients

Treatment

polyvinyl alcohol while others are made up of combinations of these or other ingredients. Dr. Paul E. Michelson, of the Scripps Clinic, in La Jolla CA writing for the Sjogren's Syndrome Foundation[53], lists thirty different brands of artificial tear drops, most of which are available without prescription.

The choice is not always easy. As Dr. Herbert Kaufman writes in *International Ophthalmological Clinic* [40] "Selecting artificial tears on a logical basis does not work." Since every patient is different, most ophthalmologists recommend a trial and error process for finding the best drops for your eyes. The optholmologist may give you samples and tell you to experiment, or your pharmacist can help you choose. There are basically three different types of artificial tears: Hypotonic (less concentrated than natural tears), plain saline, and those containing polymers. The same variety applies to the frequency of using the drops. Generally they are to be used, as needed, about four times a day for mild cases, more for severe irritations. If they are needed often, the eyes may become sensitive to preservatives in the drops and a switch would be indicated to drops utilizing a different preservative (see chart) or one of the preservative-free types. The latter should be used carefully since there is more danger of bacterial contamination which could cause infections. Generally these drops come in single-dose containers or must be kept refrigerated after opening. Often the drops are not sufficient to last through the night, in which case there are ointments available which, when placed in the eyes, will sustain the moisturizing action until morning. Some people object to these, however, as they form a thick scummy coating that causes blurry vision and must be washed out in the morning. There is also available a slow-release insert as a night application. Tiny pellets are placed under the lower lid, using a special applicator. They absorb moisture, swell, and gradually release lubricants over a long period. These pellets have some disadvantages, though, in that they are expensive and for some people who may not produce enough tears to dissolve them, the pellets may cause a feeling of something solid in the eye. I cannot use pellets so I keep a bottle of drops on the night stand by my bed. I wake frequently during the night and it's easier not to have to get up and hunt for them.

Where these methods are just not enough, other options include mucus-dispersing (mucolytic) drops, humidifiers to minimize dryness in the air, blocking of the tear drainage channels (punctal occlusion), or the use of soft contact lenses to help hold in the moisture. One enterprising inventor created a pair of glasses with a built-in reservoir of tears that run through a little trough into the eyes! [70]

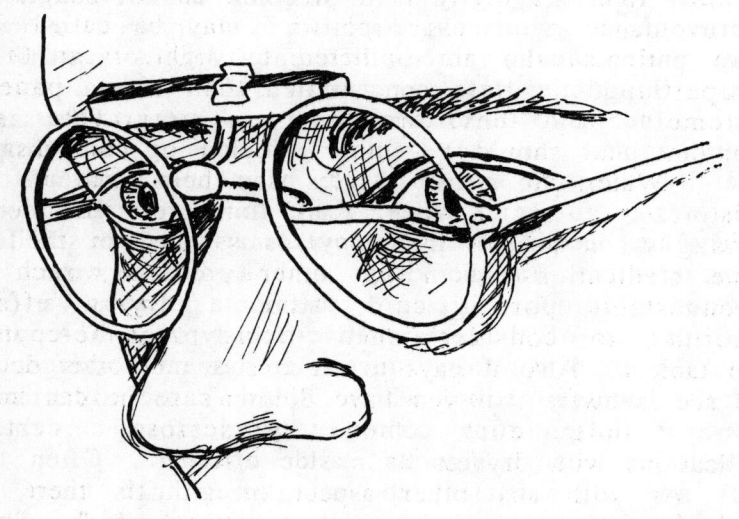

Figure 13 **Reservoir Glasses**

Punctal occlusion is used to accomplish a reverse of this idea. The puncta are ducts in the inner corner of the eyes. They are designed to allow excess fluid to drain from the eyes into the nasal ducts and eventually to the throat. For Sjogren's patients who can't afford to lose any of the precious moisture, a possible solution is to block these ducts, to retain the tears in the eyes. This can help but is sometimes only a temporary relief. None of the steps mentioned are cures, and some are

Treatment

still considered controversial or may have disadvantages. Wrap-around glasses help keep drying breezes away from the eyeballs, but are illegal to wear while driving in some states. The contact lenses prescribed as a sort of "bandage" for the eye, may cause as much irritation and infection for some people as they are designed to prevent. It is important to remember that your ophthalmologist is the only one who can properly assess the condition of your eyes and the best means of treating them. It is essential to have regular examinations, as more serious problems such as scratching of the eye covering (corneal abrasion) and infections may result from the lack of sufficient tears.

If light sensitivity is a problem, use of sunglasses and avoidance of excess exposure may be called for. Some patients who are bothered by light, wear those "wraparound" sunglasses with the side panels. Extremely dry environments can aggravate the symptoms and should be either avoided or compensated for. Watertight swim goggles can help hold in the moisture. I add a face mask for protection when working on a project that involves sawdust in the air. Some medications taken for other problems, such as decongestants for a cold, have a drying effect, important to consider when taking over-the-counter cold tablets. Also it pays to make sure any other doctor you see is aware that you have Sjogren's so he can make proper judgements about prescribing certain medications with dryness as a side effect.

As with any other aspect of arthritis there are continuing efforts to find new and better "cures". Some are genuine scientific studies and some, such as off beat diet quirks, are sheer nonsense. Be aware that any true advances come only after carefully conducted trials and investigations. Some studies now being carried out in ophthalmology include the use of topical Vitamin A; tear pumps that can be implanted directly in the eye to supply tears (maybe that man with the fancy glasses had something after all!); and a surgical transplant of salivary duct tissue to the tear gland. One esoteric idea being used is the concoction of tear drops using the patient's own blood serum. [79] These are effective but expensive and inconvenient since they use no preservatives. They must be made fresh by drawing blood periodically, and must be kept frozen. The use of gel tears and Healon (hyaluronic acid) [24] as well as drugs (Bromhexide hydrochloride) to stimulate tear production is under investigation.

In using artificial tears several precautions need to be considered. Foremost, is the need to use drops frequently. Don't wait until your eyes hurt, but establish a regular routine. Watch for signs of irritation or possible infection. Be careful not to contaminate eyes or dropper. Avoid or protect against drying environments. And be sure to discuss any changes in medication or condition with your ophthalmologist.

Dry Mouth

Many of the same concerns are applicable to the problem of a dry mouth in Sjogren's syndrome. Once again, little can be done to reverse the damage of Sjogren's, but much to alleviate and prevent. As with the eyes, the primary concern is to replace lost moisture. The obvious solution is simply to drink more water. Keeping a glass handy and just sipping on it as needed relieves the uncomfortable sensation of dryness in the mouth and throat. This is especially important when you have to talk a lot. Those long conversations on the telephone can be trying if you don't have a drink handy. Soft drinks are OK but they should be sugar-free. Not only does sugar present a danger of decay for the teeth, but it draws moisture out of the mouth tissues (by osmosis.) Often a thicker drink gives more comfort and for this tomato juice is good. My greatest temptation is to eat ice cream or drink milkshakes but this habit, carried on frequently during the day, can have disastrous results on the figure.

Sugar-free gelatin helps, but when you can't have a glass or dish of it handy, sugar-free lozenges,

Treatment 79

mints, or chewing gum can save the day. They stimulate the ailing glands to produce more saliva. Some people swear by sourball candy, so much so that one doctor has suggested that as a diagnostic tool. A piece of lemon rind or a cherry pit held in the mouth has the same potential to stimulate activity from a recalcitrant saliva gland [57], but that seems like "cruel

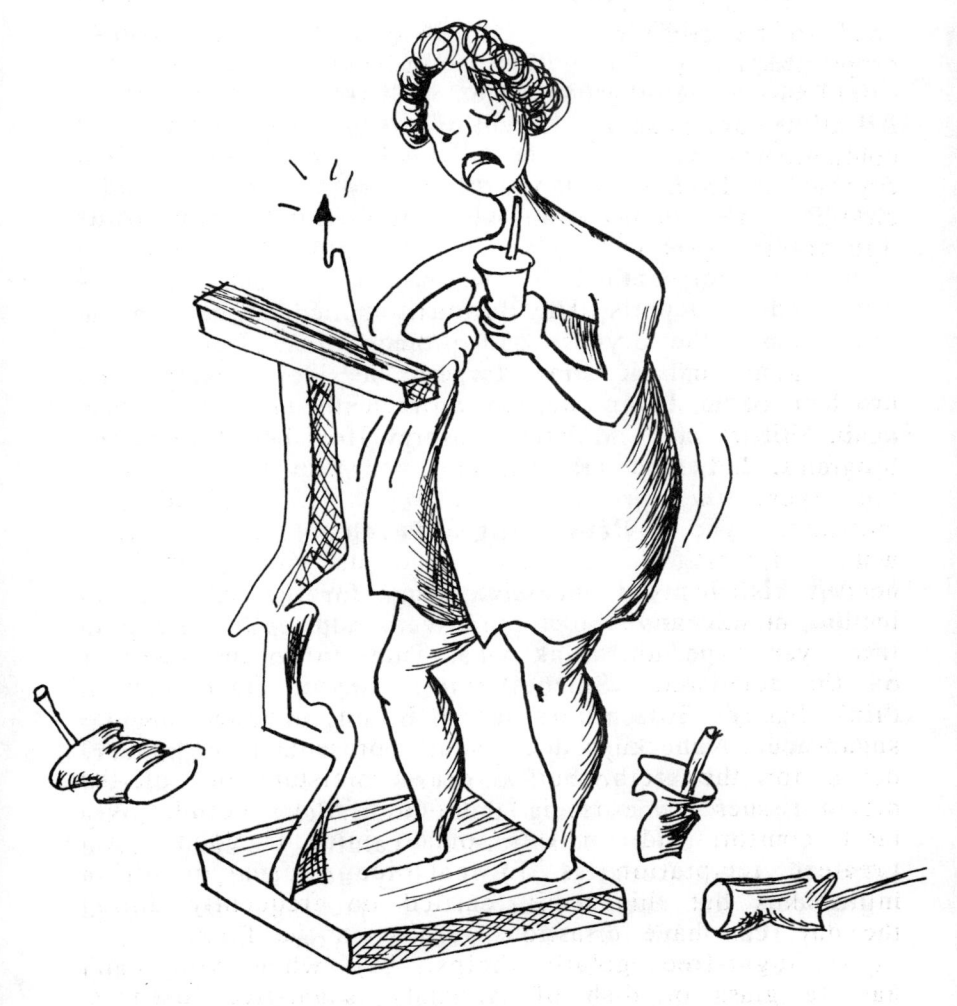

Figure **14 Too Many Milkshakes!**

and unusual punishment" to me. I always keep a glass of water (or other liquid) at my desk as I write and put one right next to my eye drops on the night stand by my bed. I also need to have some liquid with food at meals to help the mouthfuls slide along their way.

There are commercially available saliva substitutes but they are usually not entirely satisfactory. If your lips are dry or the corners of your mouth crack, they can be relieved with chapped lip sticks. Your tongue may tend to crack and therefore, be extra sensitive to spicy or acid foods.[62] I am constantly being told by "civilians" that such and such a food is "not hot at all", but even a trace of that jalapena pepper Texans love so, can burn my tender tongue. Just by natural selection I avoid citrus fruits and highly seasoned foods. Ulcers inside the mouth can sometimes be soothed by warm baking soda rinses.[92] Sara Endress reports that Borafax, applied to her lips at night, eases the dryness and protects them from getting sore. A bendable straw for her bedside drinking glass keeps it from being washed away with each sip. She uses Moistir and Moistir-10 spray for her throat and mouth just before retiring.

Protecting Teeth

In all this, I avoid excessive sugar for the sake of my teeth. If excessive sugar and teeth add up to decay in the average person, think what they do to us Sjogren's Syndrome suffers. Since the teeth are at great risk for the Sjogren's patient, it is important to have regular and frequent checkups with your dentist and to be sure he knows about your Sjogren's. There are several problems here, one being that food sticks more firmly to the teeth. For this reason, careful cleaning and flossing is essential. But beyond that, certain ingredients in normal saliva are lacking that would protect the teeth against decay. Your dentist may suggest the use of fluoride as a rinse. As in normal dental care, the best cure is prevention. This is

Treatment

especially true in Sjogren's syndrome, making one of the most emphatic points for the value of early diagnosis. Being forewarned, in this case, is being forearmed, and meticulous attention to care and cleaning may help save your teeth.

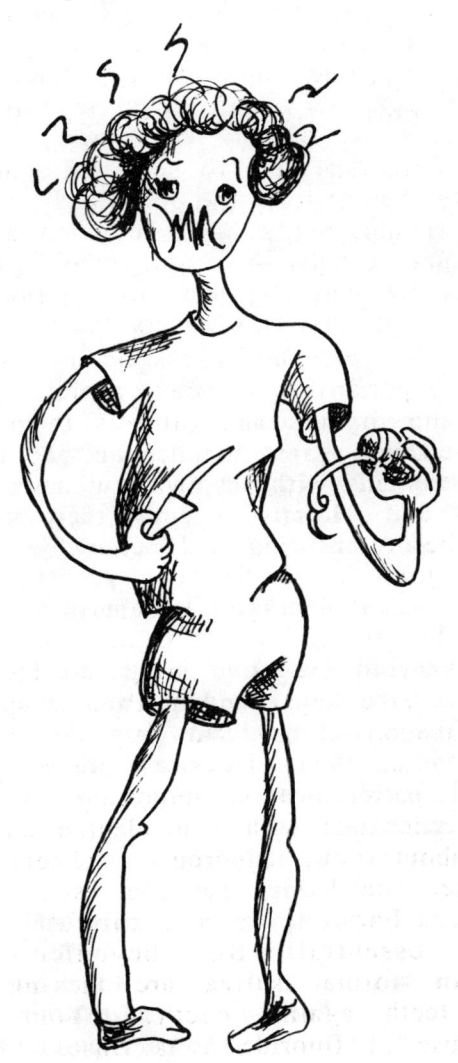

Figure 15 Lemon Peel Stimulating Saliva

Swollen Glands

The swollen salivary (parotid) glands of SS may be a cosmetic problem that the patient must simply grin and bear (difficult as that may be with such a puffy face!). If the gland damage is more severe, treatment may take the form of medication with corticosteroids, cytotoxic drugs like to those used in chemotherapy for cancer, or xray treatments.[75] As these potent procedures may have serious side effects, they are used only with caution and in severe cases. Some physicians will suggest that the disabled glands be surgically removed, but I would always ask for a second opinion on this. There is also the thought that if the glands function at all, they should be saved and encouraged.

Arthritis

The joint pains that often accompany primary Sjogren's syndrome are usually mild and can be successfully treated with aspirin or anti-inflammatory drugs (NSAIDs). These drugs do their magic in two ways. They can make you feel better by alleviating the pain of your joints, and they can prevent (or at least, slow down) the damage by helping to reduce inflammation, the source of the pain. Since these drugs can also have side effects, they must be carefully selected by your doctor in what may sometimes be a tedious and frustrating trial and error process. There is a great variety of these drugs and they have different results with different people. One type might suppress your inflammation and pain nicely, but irritate your digestive system to a dangerous degree while another might be totally ineffective for you.

The doctor can analyze benefits and possible side effects to suit your needs, but often a particular medication will require a trial run to determine if it is suitable for you. *Under no circumstances* should the patient attempt to choose his own medications or adjust them without the doctors concurrence. The information is included here only so that the patient

Treatment

SOME ANTI-INFLAMMATORY DRUGS AND THEIR POSIBLE SIDE EFFECTS

Side Effects \ Drugs	BUTAZOLIDINE	TOLECTIN	NAPROSYN	NALFON	MOTRIN	MECLOMEN	INDOCIN	FELDENE	CLINORIL	TRILISATE	ASPIRIN
INDIGESTION (GAS)	✗	✗	✗	✗	✗	✗	✗	✗	✗		✗
STOMACH IRRITATION	✗	✗	✗	✗	✗		✗	✗	✗		✗
NAUSEA	✗	✗	✗	✗	✗	✗	✗	✗	✗	✗	✗
HEARTBURN	✗	✗	✗	✗	✗	✗	✗	✗	✗		
PEPTIC ULCERS						✗					✗
CONSTIPATION								✗			
DIARRHEA						✗					
STOMACH PAIN								✗			
VOMITING										✗	✗
FLUID RETENTION	✗	✗	✗	✗	✗			✗	✗		
WEIGHT GAIN	✗										
ASCEPTIC MENINGITIS					✗						
STIFF NECK					✗						
FEVER					✗						
NERVOUSNESS							✗				
CONFUSION						✗					
ITCHING								✗			
RASH	✗	✗	✗					✗			
RINGING EARS									✗	✗	✗
HEARING LOSS										✗	✗
BLOOD THINNING											✗
LIVER DAMAGE											✗
ALLERGIES	✗	✗	✗	✗	✗		✗	✗	✗	✗	✗
RAPID BREATHING										✗	✗
LOSS OF WHITE CELLS	✗										
LOSS OF RED CELLS	✗										
HEADACHE				✗		✗		✗			

Figure 16 NSAIDs With Side Effects

may give informed consent to the regime his doctor suggests. In some cases steroids or immunosuppressive drugs may be needed but are prescribed with strong caution since they are powerful drugs.

Steroids

The term steroids includes a large category of substances created by the body or synthesized by man. Among them are cholesterol, D vitamins, bile acids, sex hormones, and the hormones secreted by the adrenal glands [77] One of the latter, cortisone, was developed as a treatment for arthritis in the '50s. The drug was hailed as a "miracle" for arthritis patients and its discoverers, Philip S. Hench and Tadeus Reichstein, were given the 1950 Nobel Prize for Medicine All over the country, swollen joints subsided and pains faded away. Arthritis sufferers were ecstatic. For a while. But after a time, it became obvious that the panacea was not without its price. In fact some side effects outweighed the benefits.

Cortisone therapy increases the patient's supply of the hormones ordinarily produced by the adrenal glands. This helps to reduce inflammation and to suppress immunological responses. Beyond the mere reduction in pain, important as that is cortisone, or the more commonly prescribed prednisone, seems to help retard the process in Sjogren's. That's the good part. But steroids have a down side that varies with the dosage and the length of time taken.

By far the majority of patients are given what are considered low doses, from 5 to 10 milligrams of prednisone per day. At this level the side effects are usually mild and can be tolerated or dealt with. Steroids may cause water retention with a resultant puffiness, especially around the face. Remember some of us suffer from puffy jaws as a result of our Sjogren's so this must be taken into consideration. An increased appetite can lead to unwelcome weight gain. Fragility of tiny blood vessels under the skin (particularly on the forearms) can cause purplish-red (but painless)

Treatment

bruises that appear at the slightest bump or scraping of the skin. When these spots fade, they leave permanent brown stains (iron deposits) under the skin in their wake. The skin itself can become thin and tear easily. In this case the result is a white scar. These problems are mostly cosmetic and a nuisance and should not necessitate stopping the therapy. Other possible problems such as dizziness, flushing, restlessness, and indigestion can occur when you first start taking prednisone but will usually go away in a couple of weeks. More major are the dangers of ulcers, depression, calcium loss, cataracts, or inflammation of the arteries(vasculitis) that can come with high dosages and/or long use. It is therefore important for the patient to be a partner with his or her physician. The doctor should carefully explain the possible disadvantages as well as the benefits from the therapy proposed. In most cases the doctor will not recommend a treatment unless the benefits will be great and the risk justified. Doctors differ in their use of steroids and if you do not fully understand or agree with your doctor's suggestions, you might get a second opinion.

One point your doctor will impress on you is that you must follow his directions explicitly. The medication must be taken exactly as indicated (ie. one in the morning and one at night, etc.) and the quantity must not be changed without his approval. Prednisone suppresses the natural activity of the adrenal glands and they tend to dry up (atrophy). If prednisone is suddenly withdrawn, the glands need time to recover so as to resume production of the hormone, hence the body would be without it for a time. To avoid this when going off the drug, one must gradually decrease the dosage, allowing the natural gland to slowly recover. In some cases (such as when undergoing surgery even for an unrelated problem), you may need a temporarily increased supply of hormones. It is important that ANY doctor who sees or treats you, knows exactly what medications you are using.

Immunosuppressives

Immunosuppressive drugs are even more powerful and dangerous than steroids and so, are used with even more caution. Only in severe, life-threatening conditions are they called for. Immunosuppressives work by attacking rapidly dividing cells. In Sjogren's, the damage is caused by proliferating (rapidly dividing) lymphocytes. When these get out of hand, immunosuppressives can help keep them in check. These are the same drugs that we hear so much about for their lifesaving role in organ transplants. When the immune system goes to work to protect the body from the alien organ the doctors have foisted upon it, immunosuppressives restrain the system, allowing the transplanted organ to function properly in its new home. The problem here is that the drugs cannot always distinguish which cells they are supposed to attack, and healthy, necessary cells may be the target. Bone marrow cells, for instance, are also rapidly-dividing cells. Increased susceptibility to infection is another danger and it is suspected (though not proven) that long term use of these drugs could cause cancer. Obviously these risks mean that the drugs must be restricted to the most severe cases.

Other treatments

Studies show that some Primary SS patients are highly subject to adverse reactions to treatment with gold salts or penicillamine. This does not seem to be true for those with secondary SS beyond what is to be expected with RA alone.

Observation

It is essential that your doctor keep close tabs on your medications. He will set a schedule for office visits which should be strictly kept. You must carefully note any changes in your condition that may possibly be side effects of the drugs, and mention them to him. The

Treatment

list and/or marked drawings will be helpful. It is sometimes hard to remember the aches and pains that plagued you yesterday when a myriad of new and different ones are competing for your attention today. It also can be trying for a doctor to listen attentively to a long vocal recital of these same complaints. A concisely stated list or a clear, simple representation on a drawing can tell him in a minute the pattern of your problems. DO NOT make any changes in your medications without first discussing them with your doctor. And feel free to call the doctor in between appointments if problems come up.

To supplement your subjective reporting, the doctor will do periodic blood workups. Many of the tests used to diagnose your Sjogren's syndrome (and any associated disease you may have) must be repeated periodically to monitor your progress. He will check on the number and volume of red and white blood cells and your sedimentation rate which measures the amount of inflammation. He may do a urinalysis to keep tabs on your kidneys. He will examine your mouth for visual evidence of dryness and irritation. There are, of course other tests to be employed for specific conditions.

Exercise

When your hips and knees hurt, the first thing you may think of is to turn on your favorite soap opera, stretch out on the sofa, and take it easy. The doctor did say get plenty of rest, didn't he? But research and good old common sense combine to tell you that kind of coddling's not the best way to treat those creaky joints. On the contrary, studies show that exercise, carefully chosen and moderately carried out, can be the best medicine. A look at the makeup of a typical joint will show you why that is true. You will notice that the joint is a closed system. That is, it is enclosed within a capsule and lubricated by the fluid created within the synovial membrane. While most tissues of the body are served by arteries that bring them essential nutrients, there are no such arteries connecting to the joint cartilage. It receives all its nourishment through the synovial fluid which must be circulated within the joint to carry out its duty of providing the nutrients and carrying off wastes. Exercise creates the movement necessary for this circulation. Furthermore, as with healthy bodies, muscles must be exercised to keep their tone and their ability to keep us in motion. The old saying "Use it or lose it." applies especially to us.[46] Evidence shows that exercise helps maintain or improve the strength of bones by slowing calcium loss.

The Arthritis Foundation divides the 109 identified types of arthritis into eight major categories,

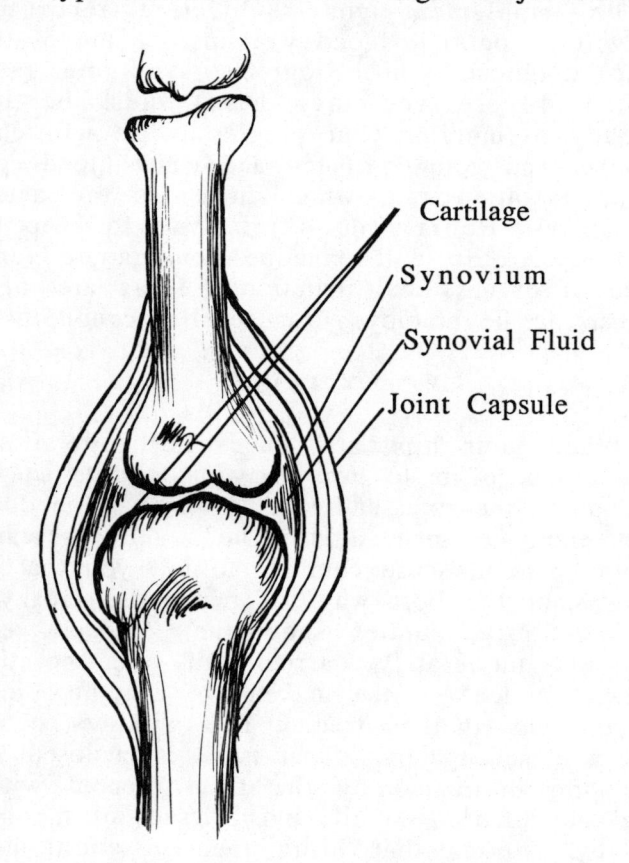

Figure 17 Joint with Synovial Capsule

Treatment

of which we need be concerned generally with only two: synovitis and muscle inflammation. Synovitis, by the Foundation"s definition, includes the conditions where an inflammation of the synovium causes the pain; the other category involves muscle inflammation. Sjogren's syndrome and its associated connective tissue diseases (rheumatoid arthritis, SLE, myositis, dermatomyositis, and scleroderma) fall into these two categories.[29]   As we have seen, exercise will help alleviate the effects of these inflammatory states.

There are other ways in which exercise is thought to help. We think we feel pain in a particular location. Swollen finger joints ache dully or our hips may protest sharply against that bending over gardening we are determined to do. But what is actually happening is that messages are being sent to our brains where the pain receptors call attention to what is happening to the knuckles. This serves an important purpose, as when we put our hands on a hot pot, the pain signal swiftly tells us to let go, before any more harm is done. Arthritis pain gives us valuable clues as to the condition of our joints and the progress of our disease. It is not advisable to try to eliminate all pain. But when we already know there's a problem, we'd just as soon have the twinges let up a bit. For this, there are natural chemicals produced in the brain, called endorphins. They act as opiates, attaching themselves to the pain receptor sites and shielding them from pain.

This is where exercise comes in. The much discussed euphoria that comes to runners after they have passed a certain pain level, comes about because the endorphins swing into action. This indicates to some researchers that the exercise itself stimulates the endorphins to do their job. Studies are being conducted to see if there are ways of artificially stimulating these chemical reactions. This could also explain the effect of activity in dissipating morning stiffness.

A serendipitous benefit of exercise is hinted at by a test of senior citizens at the University of Utah. The elderly volunteers, who had slipped into a sedentary way of life, agreed to take up a brisk aerobic conditioning program. A second bunch just put in some time doing simple stretching exercises, and a third kept right on being lazy. The studies, conducted by Dr. Robert Dustman, appear to confirm what we've thought all along, that if you keep active physically, you'll also help keep yourself more alert mentally. After only four months, tests showed significant improvement in memory, reaction time, and mental flexibility in the aerobic group and even, to the researcher's surprise, modest gains for the stretchers. Dustman was quoted in a UPI article as speculating that "those people were so out of shape that even stretching was an improvement." [26]

Type and strenuousness of an exercise program should be dictated by the nature of the patient's associated connective tissue disease, if any. Your doctor may suggest swimming or walking to help maintain flexibility of joints and muscles without placing too much stress on them. There are, according to the Arthritis Foundation's *Arthritis Helpbook*, three basic types of exercise: range of motion or stretching, strengthening, and endurance. The first type is designed to maintain flexibility by moving an individual joint through all of its natural limits in each type of motion it is expected to accomplish. The idea is to go as far as you can comfortably, and then take it just a hair further. Strengthening exercises are done by contracting the muscles without moving the joint (isometric). The isometrics can make you better able to lift and bear weight without harming your inflamed knees or elbows, etc. Endurance exercises, walking, swimming, or even dancing should be done in a smooth stressfree style to increase stamina, taking care to avoid damage to the joints. Some sports, while enjoyable as recreation, can be risky. Tennis played on a hard surface can put excessive strains on the knees, hips, and ankles, as well as causing the infamous 'tennis elbow'; bowling with a too-heavy ball can be painful for the elbows and wrists. Here again much depends on the individual. You may be experiencing stiffness in the fingers and find that typing, or even playing

Treatment 91

computer games, is good exercise. I launched my whole career as a writer because I thought typing might ward off stiffness of the fingers.

Once you start your program it is important to be as regular with it as you can. Often, you will notice that the actual walking can be painful, but this doesn't necessarily mean it's doing any harm. The Arthritis

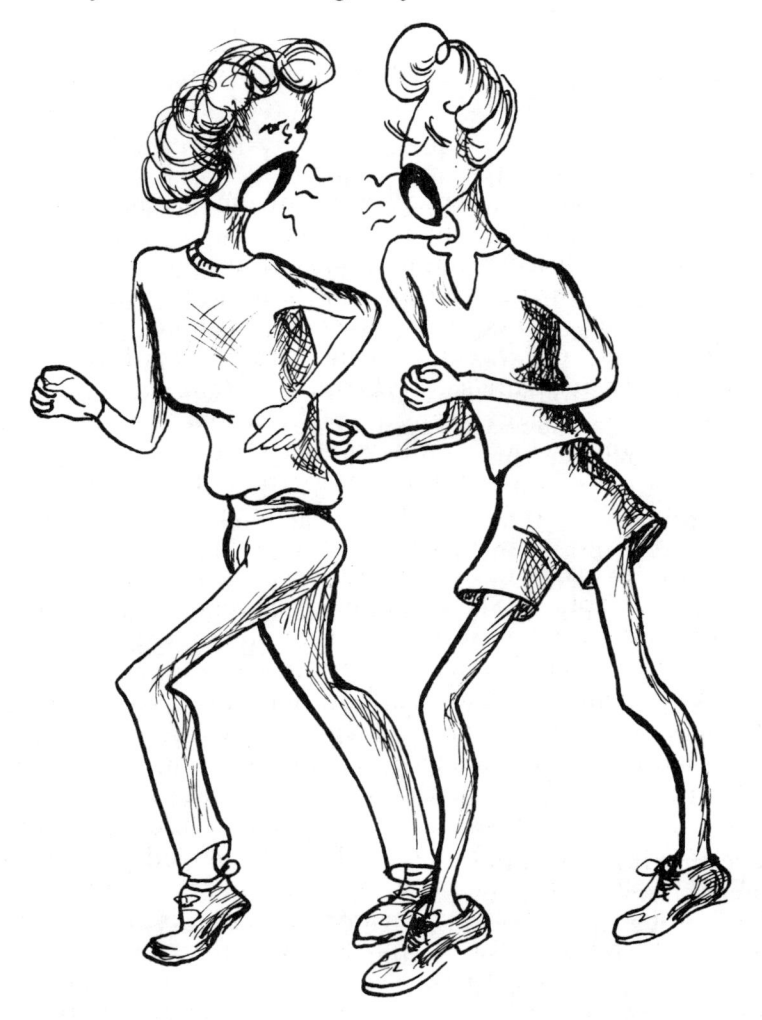

Figure 18 Walkin' and Talkin'

Foundation suggests a rule of thumb: if your exercise causes pain that persists more than two hours after you finish the exercise, you may be putting too much stress on the joint. But don't stop. Just ease up a bit. Walk a shorter distance or a little slower. Or adjust the number of days per week when you walk or swim. But consider that it may take three or four weeks before you feel any appreciable physical benefits.[19] Don't be too quick to get discouraged.

Many areas around the country now have swim exercise programs especially designed for arthritis patients and led by qualified physical therapists. I have found a regular morning walk to be the easiest program to maintain. At first, I walked alone and thought it terribly boring. I found myself making all kinds of excuses to get out of my daily walk. It was too cold out or too hot. Or I had to get the kitchen cleaned. Any excuse was a good excuse. But then I discovered a neighbor who wanted to walk, too. Now we have marked out a route (back and forth down our one block long street a specific number of times to equal the distance goal we have set for ourselves) and we walk and talk five mornings a week. We are flexible enough that obligations that interfere can keep us off a day without stopping the whole procedure. We average four days a week and this seems to bring good results. An added bonus is that we have our own little "group therapy" sessions. We can blow off steam about the frustrations of our lives to each other without having to take out the tensions on family members! We also can share the small triumphs of our lives.

I am lucky enough to have a hot tub in my home and I find it helpful to exercise each time I take a bath in it. With the wholehearted approval of my doctor, I do bicycle kicks in the water, which I have gradually increased in number over a period of time. I find that a short series of stretching exercises is good to ease the morning stiffness when I first get out of bed.

These are the things that have worked for me. I must emphasize that each person is different and will have a different level of energy and flexibility.

Treatment

Depending on the nature and extent of your arthritic involvement, you may need to work on range of motion exercises for different parts of your body. You must consult with your doctor about which exercises you should do and how strenuous they should be.

Relaxation

As with exercise, relaxation technique can provide a measure of cheap, drug free, pain relief. How many of us find ourselves gritting our already abused teeth and tensing our muscles just to get through the challenges of our days! We all know the headaches that come at the end of a long, hard day at the office, especially if the boss has chewed us out over something that wasn't our fault at all. It is not our imagination or just piling one more straw on the camel's back when we find our arthritis acting up at times like these. There is a direct cause and effect here and we can definitely do something about it.

Dianne C. Witter and Pat Hamilton Dickey describe, in <u>Arthritis Today</u> [90], special techniques we can learn to unwind those taut muscles and sooth the jangled nerves. To do this we have to be able to recognize the tension, to know in our muscles exactly how it feels, as opposed to the relaxed condition we are hoping to create. For this, psychiatrist Edmund Jacobson devised a practice he calls 'progressive relaxation'. Using special exercises, it's possible to tighten individual muscles, hold a few seconds, then release them. In kind of an 'it feels so good when you stop' approach, the pleasant feeling of relaxation that follows can ease the pain of aching joints. And a special plus is that many of the exercises can be done unobtrusively, in your office or anywhere you happen to feel the need. Witter and Dickey do suggest that you first practice them in a restful atmosphere with few distractions until you are able to ignore outside irritations. The specific exercises are detailed in Lorig and Fries' *The Arthritis Helpbook* [46] and reprinted in

the *Arthritis Today* article. [90]
Other relaxing ideas include repeating a soothing word or sound to crowd distressing thoughts out of your mind, mentally conjuring up a pleasant time or place that makes you feel at ease; or visualizing a particularly sore joint as hot and inflamed and then mentally picturing it as it cools down, allowing the pain to 'flow' out of it. You can experiment with these techniques to find what works for you and then practice until you can do them easily as needed.

Other Problem Areas

Dry Skin

Once again the major thrust of therapy for dry skin is to restore the moisture and to try to protect it from further drying out. Bathing should be limited to actual necessity. The Europeans have long derided

CREAMS AND LOTIONS
readily available at your corner store

- Nivea Cream
- Keri Lotion
- Lubriderm
- Nutraderm
- Nutraplus Cream
- Wondra
- Dermatology Formula
- Softsense
- Curel
- Neutragena
- Crisco
  (Yes, the ordinary shortening, believe it or not!)

Figure 19 Moisturizers

Americans for taking too many baths. In this case they are right, as strangely enough, soaking in water can draw the moisture out of our already dry skin. Remember as a child the way your finger tips wrinkled up like a prune after a long afternoon in the community swimming pool? This happens in a smaller way each time you wash up. Every time you bathe (and hot tubs or soaking baths can surely feel good on those aching joints!), use as little soap as possible and slather down afterwards with a good moisturizing lotion.

Sunbathing for that glorious tan should be left to others who haven't read or don't believe all the warnings of the harm it can do to even the healthiest skin. What looks lovely on an eighteen-year-old can make a 40 year old look like a senior citizen. Let's get back to the Victorian ideal of soft, unweathered skin as the ultimate beauty. Avoid the sun when possible. Cover up with long sleeves when it's not. Or if you must get right out in it, start slathering again. This time use a good sunscreen, preferably with at least a 15 rating and an added moisturizer for thorough protection.

Peripheral Problems

A distressing part of this whole mess can be the digestive upsets that seem to be our constant companions. Beginning with the need to avoid certain foods and having to explain that "it's not that I don't *like* Mexican food, it's just that it doesn't like *me*!" and running the gamut of burps and mysterious pains, we have a lot to contend with in this area. There are some ways to ease it. The most obvious is to limit or avoid foods that you know cause an upset. Acid foods such as citrus fruits or tomatos may be the villains. Or highly spiced foods. Chinese food, which I love, seems to give me a lot of trouble. Some people suffer from lactose intolerance and should be careful of dairy products. Naturally, you should consider the important elements these foods contain (such as calcium, vitamins, and proteins) and find other sources for them.

Antacids with anti-gas ingredients or acid-inhibiting drugs may be prescribed by your doctor, but should be used only under his supervision. Dr. Katz has observed that antacids are useless against the indigestion of Sjogren's syndrome that is originally caused by a *lack* of acid. This is what happens when SS causes the hydrochloric acid-producing glands to atrophy (literally dry up and fail to secrete enough acid). Similarly, inflammation of the stomach lining itself is not soothed by antacids. In other patients the heartburn may be brought on by excess acid as a result of decreased dilution by saliva. In this case, water alone may bring welcome relief. If refluxing (rising of stomach contents into esophagus) is a problem, it helps to sleep with head elevated. Just putting something under the head of your mattress to raise it about 4 inches achieves this. A few old books you are tired of having around, will do. Cut out those heavy bedtime snacks and turn down burp-producing goodies like onions or baked beans. As a matter of fact, simply remembering not to overeat at any one time will make a difference. But be sure to discuss your digestive problems with your doctor and follow his advice.

Vaginal Dryness

In Chapter 2, I promised help for this personal aspect of Sjogren's syndrome. As with all the other symptoms, there is no quick and easy solution. But there are ways to ease the discomfort and avoid the more serious consequences. We have seen that dryness can come from a lot of different causes. Infections, allergies, irritating chemicals, stress, some surgeries, menopause, childbirth, and even hurried sex can be suspected. [71] Allergies and chemicals, which include soap, perfumed douches or bubble baths, perspiration, detergents, bath powder, fabric softeners, synthetic fabrics themselves and even plain tap water (filled with minerals) can be the most common villains. But they are the most easily remedied. Just say no. To all of those things, you ask? That may not be necessary. Here there is a principal of mechanical trouble shooting that applies. To find out what in particular is bothering you, eliminate one thing at a time. Try just

Treatment

soaking in water with about a tablespoon of vinegar instead of using soap. Use unscented powders. Wear all cotton panties for a while. Experiment with different brands of laundry detergent. One at a time. Then, if the irritation eases, you will know precisely what was causing it. Or if none of those things are guilty, press on to other aspects. Just do some detective work. Are you over tired? Worried about your job? Just feeling irritated at the world? All of these things can slow down the vaginal secretions and leave you dry and uncomfortable. If none of these are the culprit, you will need to work with your doctor, first checking through all the medications you are taking to see if any of them are making you dry. They could be the same ones that affect other parts of your body. He may suggest some changes or he may advise using lubricants. Dr. Sheehy suggests avoiding vaseline. He recommends Lubrin, cold cream and sex, not necessarily in that order. The latter, he says is "not only beneficial psychologically, but can help restore vaginal lubrication and elasticity, preventing loss of support ot the bladder." He adds that when having sex, that pleasurable foreplay serves a definite purpose. Without it the glands may not be properly stimulated to provide lubrication. And that, in turn, can make sexual fulfillment iffy. That's when you need to ask for the loving co-operation of your partner.

Menopause and childbirth related discomfort may be due to a hormone imbalance and this can be checked. When your doctor takes a Pap smear, he can also arrange to test your estrogen level, and if needed, you can take tablets to raise your level. This must be done cautiously and your doctor will probably also prescribe progesterone to ward off the danger of cancer of the uterus. If the Bartholin's glands themselves are the root of the trouble, your gynecologist can unplug them.

A Word to the Wise

On one trip to my doctor's office I happened to

wear a lovely copper bracelet my husband had brought me as a souvenir from a trip west. My doctor was upset, until I hastily assured him I expected no magical cures from the bangle. The copper-bracelet-as-arthritis-cure gimmick is relatively innocent, and, in fact, it can be fun to adopt a tongue-in-cheek 'let's cover all the bases' approach once in a while. However, there are, and have been as long as people have had the 'rheumatiz', shady entrepreneurs who will peddle anything a gullible public will buy as a sure-fire cure for all your aches and pains. Dr. James F. Fries reports, in *Arthritis: A Comprehensive Guide*, [29] that arthritis patients spend hundreds of millions of dollars per year chasing the rainbows of quick cures. My bracelet was inexpensive and had its own beauty and intrinsic value, but the villains of this story are the predators who will charge just as much as their victims are willing to pay for the wonderful promise of relief. The spectrum ranges from books that promote a quirky diet to 'cleanse your system', to elaborate clinics that propose to cure a marvelous variety of ills with a 'scientific' new treatment or drug. Large numbers of people travel across the border to Mexico or to other foreign countries to take 'miracle' pills which our admittedly cumbersome FDA process prohibits in the US. Among the exotic cures discussed by Dr. Fries are bee sting venom, flu shots, cod liver oil, acupuncture, acupressure, and frequent enemas. The cod liver oil is used to 'oil' the joints! Acupuncture, whatever benefits it may have, has been shown to have no effect on arthritis and is not used for that purpose even in China. Those prohibited pills are either being tested to prove their safety and efficacy, or have already been proven to lack those qualities. In spite of glorious claims, for instance, the industrial solvent DMSO has not been proven effective for arthritis, although it is approved for urologists to use as a treatment for interstitial cystitis. The legal pain-pills advertised ubiquitously on our TV as being specially formulated for arthritis, are no better than the plain varieties of aspirin, only more expensive.

Treatment

The wonderful world of quackery has thrived through the ages. Probably as long as there have been human ailments. The record goes back a long way. In 1856 a well preserved spine from a Neanderthal man was found, cruelly distorted by arthritis. Eric Jameson records, in his *The Natural History of Quackery* [37] a story originally published in the *Northern Imposter* in 1786 of "the Late, Celebrated, Dr. Rock", as follows:

'He was standing one day at his door on Ludgate Hill, when a real doctor of Physic passed, who had learning and abilities, but whose modesty was the true cause of his poverty.

'"How comes it," says he to the quack, "that you without education, without skill, without the least knowledge of science, are enabled to live in the style you do? You keep your town house, your carriage, and your country house: whilst I, allowed to possess some knowledge, have neither, and can hardly pick up a subsistence!"

"Why look ye," said Rock smiling, "how many people do you think have passed since you asked me the question?"

'"Why," answered the Doctor, "perhaps a hundred."

'"And how many out of those hundred, think you, possess common sense?"

'"Possibly one," answered the Doctor.

'"Then," said Rock, "that one comes to you: and I take care of the other ninety-nine."'

Jameson records the story of another physician, working a hundred years earlier, named Paracelsus, who proposed an ingenious 'cure' for disease. His treatment involved a magnet impregnated with 'mummy', preferably one made from a criminal who had been hanged, as from these there was a 'gentle siccation that expungeth the watery humor'. After sowing some 'seeds that have a congruity with the disease', the practitioner was to rub the 'mummified' magnet over the affected parts of the patient and plunge it into the earth near the planted seeds. As the seeds germinated and grew, the disease would be drawn out of the patient and he would be cured. 'Forget the old classical medicine,' Paracelsus told his students, 'and follow my doctrines.'

By the year that twisted old cave man was found,

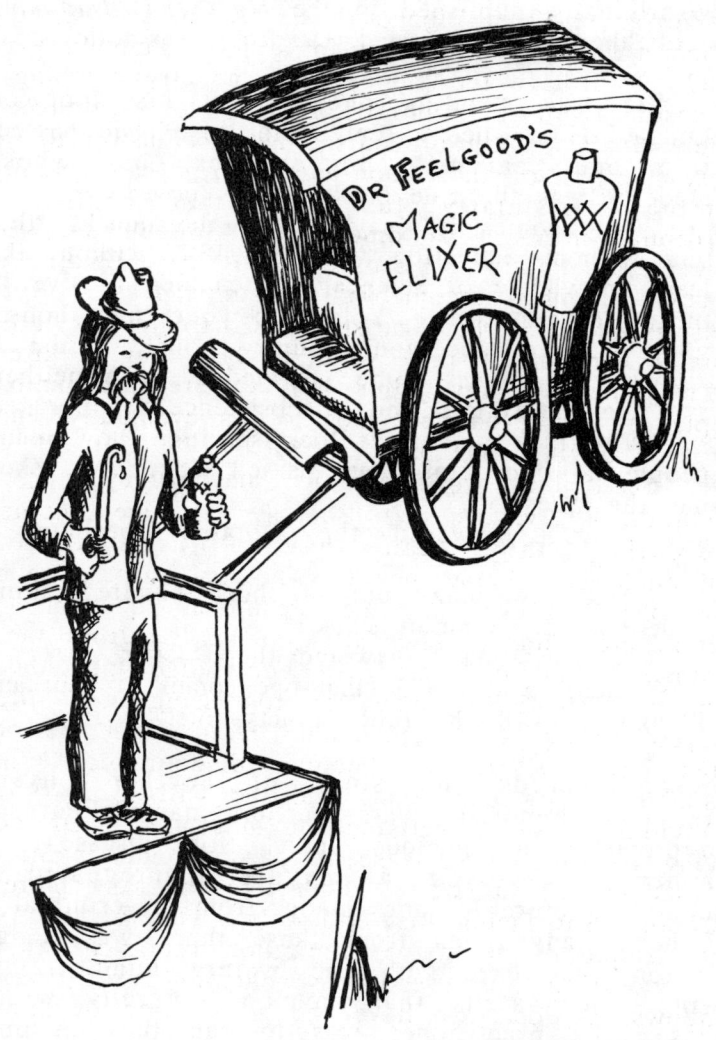

Figure *20* **Quack Selling "Joint Oil"**

Treatment

living Americans with the same painful problem had an astounding 1500 different nostrums to choose from. Most were blends of alcohol, narcotics, or a variety of toxic substances added to flavored sugarwater. Even today, according to the Consumers' Union's *Report on Fake Health Claims, Worthless Remedies, and Unproved Therapies*,[27] 32 million arthritic Americans spend 950 million a year on their quest for relief. You may say, so what? If I have the money, why not try anything, just in case? Even a mummified magnet, if there's any chance at all? Well, of course, the first answer to that is safety. Some of those non-legal 'cures' can actually be harmful, particularly fad diets that neglect vital nutritional needs. Some medications can seriously affect other body systems, or are just plain toxic. Especially under uncontrolled circumstances. But Dr. Fries points out that most quack treatments are not actually harmful or they wouldn't last long. After all, we may have creaky joints but we are not dumb. If people are being harmed, most of us eventually find out and quit buying that one.

So if they won't hurt us, maybe they <u>will</u> help. It's worth a try, we say. But if they are not harmful medically, they can have other unpleasant consequences. Some people who try these treatments, turn their backs on the traditional methods their doctors are using. Thus they are not getting the best treatment that our medical knowledge provides for them. The disease may be progressing in a direction that could have been prevented. And when the phoney cures don't work, we become discouraged with all treatment, losing confidence and the will to carry on.

Obviously not a satisfactory situation. Of course, having to say our disease is chronic and incurable is not satisfactory either. I don't like that any more than you do. But facing that and doing what we can within that (temporary, we hope) limitation is far better than wasting our resources chasing those slippery rainbows. Besides, we have the satisfaction of knowing

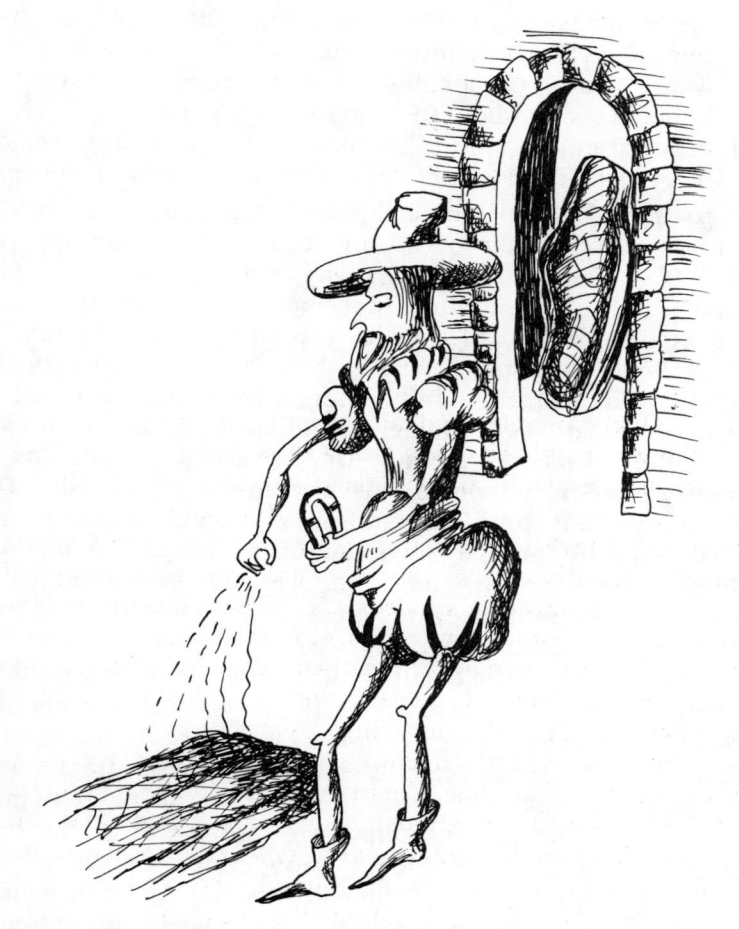

Figure 21 Paracelsus Planting 'Mummified' Magnet Seeds

that those sleazy con-men cannot succeed, if we don't buy.

None of this applies to the legitimate efforts of dedicated scientists to find the solutions for us. Some of these stories will be told in the chapter on research, and may, truthfully, seem much more exciting than even the most exotic of the snake oil merchants' claims!

Chapter 7

Research

One constant refrain heard in my letters from SS Chapter members goes like this: "I hope they are doing some research about this disease!" Well, the good news is, they definitely are. Eminent doctors and scientists literally around the world are working diligently to pry open the secrets of cause and effect that create Sjogren's syndrome. That has not always been true. For many years, as many of us are well aware, SS has been an orphan disease, hardly even earning recognition as a *disease*, but just considered a rare combination of annoying symptoms.

But in recent decades, and particularly in the eighties, the quest has finally taken hold. Specialists around the world in almost every discipline that enters into the Sjogren's puzzle are conducting experiments and following lines of study about the causes, course, and treatment of SS. Leading the field is Dr. Norman Talal, currently working through the Division of Clinical Immunology and Arthritis at the University of Texas Health Science Center in San Antonio, Texas where he is Professor of Medicine and Microbiology and Chief of the Division.[74] He is also Chief of the Section of Clinical Immunology and Arthritis at Audie L. Murphy Veterans Administration Hospital. Dr. Talal is co-editor, along with Dr. H. M. Moutsopoulos and Dr. S. S. Kassan, of *Sjogren's Syndrome, Clinical and Immunological Aspects*, a state-of-the-art medical textbook published in the fall of 1987.[80]

After medical school, internship, residency, and post-doctoral training in medicine at Columbia University, Dr. Talal spent a year as a research fellow at the Institut de Recherches Scientifiques sur le Cancer in Paris. Following that he was a clinical associate and then Senior Investigator at the National Institute of Arthritis and Metabolic Diseases from 1962 to 1971. His first paper on Sjogren's syndrome, published in 1968 in the American Journal of Medicine, is regarded as a classic. In 1972, as a professor of medicine at the University of California, San Francisco, he enlisted the help of Dr. Troy E. Daniels and Dr. Bruce Ostler to establish the Sjogren's Syndrome Clinic at that University. Dr. Talal also served as Chief of the Clinical Immunology and Arthritis Section of San Francisco's VA Hospital. In 1981, he left there to come to the University of Texas. He is chairman of the medical advisory board of the SS Foundation, director of an Arthritis Foundation Clinical Center, Principal Investigator of an NIH Training Grant in Rheumatology, and chairman of the Honorary Membership Committee of the American Rheumatism Association. [74]

An authority on immunoregulation, Dr. Talal has published an extensive array of papers and a chapter on SS in D.J. McCarty's *Arthritis and Allied Conditions* and is currently engaged in research aimed at a better understanding of immune response mechanisms and autoimmunity. He is particularly interested in discerning the cause and development of autoimmune diseases. From the Health Science Center, he directs the Multipurpose Arthritis Center and its special multi-disciplinary clinic devoted to patients with Sjogren's syndrome. Hopes are high that what is learned there will lead to the development of new drugs capable of modulating the erring immune system at the root of the bewildering problems of Sjogren's syndrome and the other autoimmune diseases. Other scientists at San Antonio are studying T cells, the activation of

Research

lymphocytes, and the relationship of nutrition, aging, and sex hormones to the immune responses.

Similar study programs are being carried out at other centers in the United States and in other countries around the world. American researchers include Dr. Philip Fox whose work at the National Institute of Dental Research, NIH in Bethesda, Maryland, focuses on ways to relieve and treat the oral components of SS. At the University of California San Francisco Sjogren's Syndrome Clinic, under Dr. Daniels and Dr. Ostler, with Dr. John P. Whitcher, patients are referred by dentists, ophthalmologists and rheumatologists for treatment. Dr. Daniels, a dentist, is especially interested in studying the immune system diseases of the mouth and salivary glands.[2,3]

Dr. Frank C. Arnett, Director of Rheumatology Division, University of Texas Health Science Center/Houston, is studying the incidence of neonatal SLE with mothers carrying the anti-Ro (SS-A) antibody, a Sjogren's syndrome marker.

At the Rheumatology and Clinical Immunology Divisions of the Department of Medicine of Johns Hopkins University in Baltimore, Maryland, Dr. Elaine Alexander and her colleagues are currently investigating the effects of SS on central and peripheral nervous system disorders, and focussing on the genetics of SS and lupus. Dr. Douglas Jabs at the Wilmer Ophthalmological Institute of Johns Hopkins searches for ways to relieve our dry eyes.

Dr. Susumi Sugai, who traces his interest in Sjogren's syndrome to his days working with Dr. Talal in the San Francisco clinic, is now working in Ishikawa, Japan, studying possible differences in genetic factors between Japanese and Caucasian SS patients. Official studies were conducted from 1976 to 1980 by an SS research committee, headed by Dr. Tadashi Ofuji (president of Okayama University in 1987) with Dr. Shoji Miyawaki of the University's 3rd Department of Internal Medicine, and sponsored by the Japanese Health and Welfare Ministry.

Dr. Jan Ulrik Prause, an associate professor in the Eye Pathology Institute at Denmark's University of Copenhagen, began studying Sjogren's syndrome in 1972. Beginning with a small group of scientists who were personal friends, the research effort grew to include investigators from other parts of Denmark, from Sweden, and from Norway to evolve into an all-Scandinavia Sjogren's group. They established a journal to standardize the way they report their medical findings and then carried that idea even further into the contemporary world of medical research. They are currently compiling a centralized computer database. It will contain medical information gained from SS patients throughout the Scandinavian countries, which will be useful in creating wide based studies in many aspects of Sjogren's syndrome with the shortest possible time required to accumulate large amounts of information. This will allow the same sets of tests to be used in many studies, creating an exchange of knowledge, and avoiding the duplication of effort while at the same time putting the available research dollars to maximum use.

In Greece, studies by Dr. H. M. Moutsopoulos, Dr. S. H. Constantopoulos, and their colleagues in the Department of Internal Medicine at the University of Ioannina's Medical School have investigated the areas of lung disease and kidney and gastrointestinal problems in Sjogren's syndrome. Salivary gland involvement has also been studied by the team.

Dr. Moutsopoulos says he is another one of the doctors "introduced to the fascinating spectrum of Sjogren's syndrome by Norman Talal in the beginning of the '70s." He worked with SS patients initially in San Francisco and at the United States National Institute of Health (1976-1980), then returned to his native Greece. There his Immunology Laboratory for clinical (diagnostic) and research work follows over 100 patients with primary and secondary Sjogren's.

Others are carrying out a wide variety of studies in the People's Republic of China, Holland, France, and the Soviet Union.

Chronology

Dedicated doctors have been concerned with these studies for several decades, publishing findings on lymphoma in SS as early as 1963. Martin Shearn, as an Associate Professor of Medicine at the University of California at San Francisco, wrote his book, *Sjogren's Syndrome* in 1971. Yet the real momentum has picked up only in the 80s. Drs. Pavlidis, Karsh, and Moutsopoulos proposed designations of primary and secondary Sjogren's syndrome in 1981, based on studies of clinical, serological, and immunological differences between SS alone and SS with an associated connective tissue disease.[58] Manthorpe, Frost-Larsen, Isager, & Prause also favored the introduction of the terms Primary and Secondary.[49]

In May 1986, Dr. Prause joined Dr. Rolf Manthorpe of Sweden's Lund University to host the first International Seminar on Sjogeren's Syndrome in Copenhagen. Researchers gathered from countries as far separated as the United States, Greece, and Japan to present the findings of their individual investigations. A major achievement of the conference was the discussion of the varied diagnostic criteria then in use and efforts to come to a concensus for worldwide standardization of these criteria.

Arthritis

In the broader field of arthritis research, investigators are taking several different approaches. Immunologists tracking the cellular basis of inflammatory diseases are now carrying their studies on to the molecular level and are hoping to identify points in the process that may be blockable with new drugs. Researchers are looking for ways to "turn off" the defective genes that trigger auto-immune responses. Dr. Michael B. Oldstone of the Research Institute of Scripps Clinic in La Jolla, California is using a virus to inhibit the autoimmune action of a lymphocyte in laboratory mice.[61] Clues are being found to the genetic factors involved which will help doctors anticipate the development of disease. Better knowledge of the mechanics of joint movement and interaction will lead to more understanding of the beneficial exercises and ways to limit damage to bones and tissues, while studies of the chemical structure of cartilage is expected to yield progress in preventive medication in this area. Other researchers are looking for new ways to use existing drugs and procedures such as irradiation and a treatment known as plasmapharesis, which aims at cleansing offending substances from the blood.

Many of these studies, being carried out with special regard to rheumatoid arthritis, lupus, and or other autoimmune diseases will affect the work on Sjogren's syndrome, and some data gained from SS work impact the entire field of immunology.

Pie in the Sky

The fact that SS and some other autoimmune diseases (particularly SLE) appear most inclined to attack women, and especially women in the childbearing years, inspired researchers to look for a connection. Dr Talal reported in 1978 on studies that seem to indicate that female sex hormones (estrogen) can exacerbate autoimmune diseases while male hormones (androgens) tend to suppress them. Alfred Steinberg, another scientist whose research interest started in Dr. Talal's laboratory, and others at the National Institute of Health (NIH) observed that male hormones tend to favor the suppressor T cells while female hormones encourage the production of helper T cells, which we learned earlier stimulate the activities of both the killer T cells and the antibody producing B cells.[54] There is some evidence that SLE patients may benefit from androgen treatment (Danazol).[78] Dr. S. Ansar Ahmed is conducting ongoing studies in San

Antonio into the control of immunity and autoimmunity by sex hormones.[76]

Pilocarpine, a drug being tested by Dr. Fox at Bethesda, gives hope of being able to stimulate saliva production. Pilocarpine is presently used as an ingredient in some prescription eye drops.[59]

Bromhexine is a drug that increases bronchial secretions and reduces viscosity. Produced commercially in Europe as Bisolvon™, bromhexine comes from an old Indian folk herb medicine that has been extracted from the plant *Adhatoda vasica*, for more than 500 years.[52] Dr. Prause in Denmark has studied the use of bromhexine, and it is used routinely in Europe for bronchitis as well as to improve tear and saliva secretions.[65] It has not yet been approved for use in the United States. Positive results have been seen in tests on laboratory mice and, additionally, the drug seems to lessen the destruction of tissue by deranged immune cells. Because of its long history, the drug is not patentable, which puts it into the class of 'orphan drugs' (those whose lack of profitability makes them impractical for American drug firms to produce). Tests to satisfy the Food and Drug Administration's strict safety and effectiveness standards are costly but Boehringer-Ingelheim Pharmaceuticals Inc, a US company, is initiating Investigational New Drug studies to make the drug legal here.[31]

Drs. Prause and Manthorpe have also conducted placebo studies on another plant-derivative drug. A fatty acid (gamma-linolenic acid or GLA) derived from evening primrose oil is being suggested as a means of promoting the body's production of prostaglandins used to fight infection and inflammation.[52] GLA supplies chemicals needed to produce prostaglandin EI which helps regulate the inflammatory process. According to Dr. James Sciubba of the Long Island Jewish Medical Center, evening primrose oil, manufactured as Efamol "is considered safe and ... worth trying" He adds that is must be used at least a month for any benefits. The Scandinavian tests indicated that those patients experienced a lessening of the universal tiredness that accompanies SS. However, Dr. Frank Arnett of the University of Texas Health Science Center at Houston, describes it as "an unproven remedy".

In Greece, Prof. Moutsopoulos and his associates have conducted clinical trials of Cyclosporin A, another plant-related substance, but the results were disappointing. Although a decrease in destructive lymphocytes was seen, little actual improvement in the patients' condition was observed.[25]

Studies of Vitamin A in eye drops have been controversial. Although the vitamin is used in Europe, there have been no proven effects when taken internally, and tests of its topical use (directly in the eyes) have not used the 'blind' control in which neither doctor nor patient knows who is getting what treatment. Because people tend to want good results, Dr. Prause comments, "These all turn out positive." One such test, carried out in 1984 by Dr. Scheffer Chuei-Goong Tseng at the Massachusetts Eye and Ear Infirmary of Harvard Medical School, followed 22 dry eye patients, some of whom had been diagnosed as having Sjogren's syndrome. All were selected because conventional methods had not helped them, and all reported improvement in tear production, vision, and relief from dryness, irritation, and light sensitivity after treatment with a Vitamin A ointment. At a Science Writers Seminar in Ophthalmology, Dr. Tseng stated that he observed reversal of damaged tissue and regeneration of goblet (mucus secreting) cells.[84]

Fortunately for us Sjogren's patients, the negative or questionable results of some experiments cannot deter these investigators from pursuing other avenues and new findings are being rapidly made. Much new information will have been uncovered even before this book can be completed; and with the increased awareness and concern by researchers, health professionals and patients themselves, progress is bound to be made.

Chapter 8

Help

Prognosis

For most patients SS has a benign course, that is, its multiple symptoms provide only varying degrees of inconvenience or discomfort. But that does not mean, as some medical practitioners have felt, that it should be taken lightly. When I recently remarked to my pharmacist that there ought to a specialty known as "exocrinology", he replied that the exocrine glands were not considered important! You have only to have them fail to function properly to realize how far from the mark that comment is. True, the vast majority of Sjogren's patients never experience any life-threatening difficulties but the problems can certainly be lifeSTYLE threatening. The very fact that a Sjogren's patient quite often shows no visible signs of illness, can cause major misunderstandings among families and co-workers. The need for rest periods when your flag suddenly droops is rarely obvious to companions. A dilemma occurs for the patient who doesn't want to be a complainer and yet has a need for some people close to her to understand her situation. I have always had a philosophy that says if you have a problem, (the illness) that's one problem; but if you moan and complain about it, you then have two problems! You and your friends and family have to work through the unpleasantness of your misery before anyone can react positively to the illness. Instead, you have to accept and calmly discuss some limitations with whatever good will you can muster. Those around you need to be aware of those limitations if you are to function well.

The inconveniences of Sjogren's generally can be handled by the methods used to treat the symptoms, and preventive vigilance. For the latter purpose, the earliest possible diagnosis is vital.

In particular, there is an antibody labeled Ro (SSA) in the blood of some women with Sjogren's syndrome. Because this antibody may be associated with heart problems in newborn infants [12,88] researchers are suggesting that women with SS who become pregnant or are considering having a baby, should ask their doctors about testing for this antibody. The infants may have NLE (neonatal lupus erythematosis) which involves a skin rash that appears at birth but usually heals spontaneously along with a more-serious possibility of heart blockage.

Some patients may have RA factors without having RA, or antinuclear antibodies without having SLE.[7] More-serious consequences can occur, including the extra-glandular manifestations previously discussed: psuedo lymphomas (benign), lymphomas (malignancies), or Waldenstrom's macroglobulinemia (excessive growth of plasma cells).

Support Resources

Bernice Kapalin, forced by corneal ulcers to leave her job, feels 'like a freak because so many people, including some nurses she knows, never heard of SS.' Helen Ruhl, who writes that she is "learning to live with her SS", laments that she knows no one else who has it. "I am," she says, "a rare bird."

Prognosis/Support 113

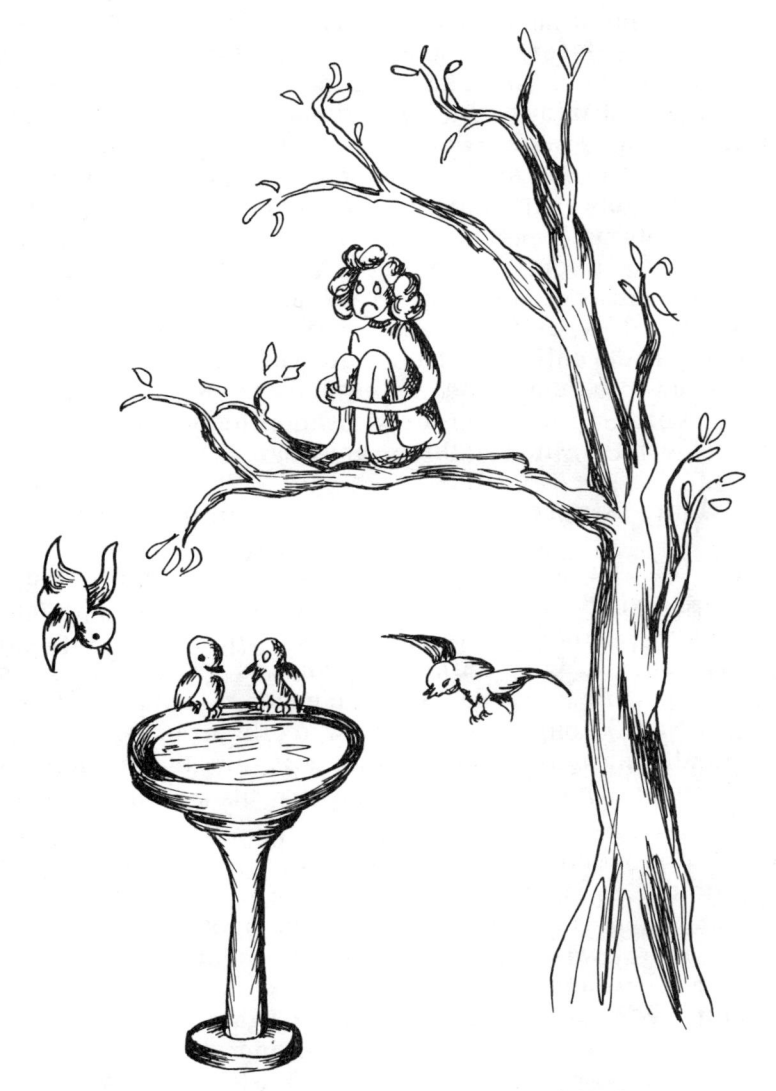

Figure 22 **The Rare SS Bird**

As we have seen, that may not be so, according to the doctors investigating SS. But loneliness among an invisible crowd is one of the commonplaces of SS patients. There are hundreds of stories of women with sad tales of going from doctor to unsympathetic doctor and feeling more and more lonely and depressed all the time. Please forgive me, I know there are men involved, too, but since SS appears to be partial to women, and there is this unfortunate stereotype of the unfulfilled housewife who turns to hypochondria for solace, most of the stories I've heard come from women. They have gone for months or years being told "you are an emotional woman", "go home, put your contacts in, and forget about it." or "it's all part of menopause." Even after you get a diagnosis of SS, it seems no one's ever heard of it and you feel very much alone. Often husbands and children have grown tired of hearing about your problems and it seems, as Kapalin put it, hardly worth going grocery shopping and cooking when "I can't taste anything anyway."

The Sjogren's Syndrome Foundation

If you fit into that lonely category, take heart. There are others who understand how you feel. And they have banded together to form a support organization. Originally known as The Moisture Seekers, the organization was founded by Elaine Harris of Great Neck, Long Island in New York in 1983.

It all started when Elaine was in the office of allergist Dr. Paul Lang complaining of a stuffy head, clogged up ears, and swollen glands.[44] When she added a dry mouth to the list, Dr. Lang began to suspect her problem was not allergy but Sjogren's syndrome. In those days having SS was even more lonely than now as there was little information about this peculiar malady and no one around to share symptoms.

Out of sheer frustration, Elaine, with the encouragement of her doctors at Long Island's Jewish Medical Center and the help of the Arthritis Foundation, set about to remedy both problems. She arranged the first meeting of The Moisture Seekers in December of 1983.[32] Fourteen Sjogren's syndrome patients with 11 of their supportive relatives met to

hear Dr. James Sciubba explain their mysterious disorder.
   Established for the sole purpose of getting SS patients together, to increase awareness, and to promote research, the group grew into the present Sjogren's Syndrome Foundation, Inc.   Elaine Harris still serves as its president and guiding light.   By May 1987 there were 23 chapters in the United States, one in England and one in Japan. At that time there were 13 more chapters being formed in the US and one in Canada. The rate of growth is such that by the time this goes to press there will surely be many more chapters in cities across the country and around the world.   If there still is not one near you, you can find help in forming one by contacting the Foundation. (Write to Anita Shehi, 7314 East Papago Drive, Scottsdale AZ 85257)   Meetings for most chapters are held monthly with leading physicians and researchers as speakers. Topics range from specifics about the care and feeding of dry eyes to discussions of the problems of coping with chronic disease.   Speakers' specialties include dentistry, immunology, gynecology, dermatology, and many more areas that can be affected by SS. Other subjects discussed range from the oral health care program recommended by the National Institute, and tips on what to do about a dry or stuffy nose. At least one chapter (Baltimore) video-tapes these seminars and makes the tapes available to members at cost. The New York Chapter heads the organization in three rooms of the Harris' Long Island home where Ms. Harris edits and produces the Foundation's monthly newsletter, *The Moisture Seekers*.   This contains news of the chapters and individual members as well as reprints of talks given by speakers. Copies of the newsletter on specific subjects are available from foundation headquarters. The Foundation is served by a Medical Advisory Board which, in 1987, included Norman Talal, M. D., Chairman; Mark Abelson, M.D.; Steven Carsons, M.D.; Troy Daniels, D.D.S.; Vincent P. deLuise, M.D.; Herbert S. Diamond, M.D.; R. Linsy Farris, M.D.; Richard Furie, M.D.; Jeffrey Gilbard, M.D.; John Greenspan, B. D. S.; Robert A.

Greenwald, M.D.; Howard Kerpen, M.D.; H. Clifford Lane, M. D.; Irwin Mandel, D.D.S.; Athena Papas, D.M.D. Ph. D.,James J. Sciubba, D.M.D. Ph.D.; Harry Spiera, M.D.; and Ira J. Udell, M.D.   These doctors are all actively researching Sjogren's syndrome or working with SS patients.

The Sjogren's Syndrome Foundation is a grass roots organization created and continued by the very people it serves. This can cause problems when you realize that fatigue, often extreme fatigue, is a major and almost universal symptom of SS. It's hard to be a mover and shaker when you really feel like crashing most of the time, and the simplest daily chores can seem monumental at times.

When Anita Shehi, in Phoenix Arizona, was diagnosed as having Sjogren's syndrome, her rheumatologist gave her a copy of the Arthritis Foundation's SS booklet. Anita looked for more information in her local library but found only the not too comforting news that the odds for getting SS were one in two thousand. Still curious, she tried to delve deeper by visiting the local hospital's medical library. There she was refused access because she was not a medical professional! Desperate for some comfort, she wrote to the 'Moisture Seekers', whose address is listed in the Arthritis Foundation booklet. Elaine Harris' response was to urge her to start a support group in Phoenix and the first Arizona chapter was born . From a beginning with six or seven people that group has grown to a healthy 80 members. Now Anita helps others who want to start local chapters.

Sara Endress is a gutsy lady who enjoys living in Tucson, Arizona, in spite of her doctor's comments that the dry climate is unfriendly to SS patients. At 68, she has joined a health club, is active in aerobics, takes a 'splash dance' class three times a week, and swims in the heated pool at her mobile home park. Her biggest problem with Arizona's climate is avoiding the ever-present airconditioning most of her neighbors can't live without. Sara founded the Tucson chapter of the SS Foundation. The group's twelve members began

Prognosis/Support

meeting late in 1986 and are carrying on the work Sara began. While Sara keeps active on her mobile park board of directors, and her church, she says trying to arrange for the SS meetings month after month had her feeling "a little pushed". As a widow who takes care of her own car and home, plus working in her small garden (I *do* do windows", she says), she finds her time and energy precious. Her dry and irritated eyes force her to limit activities like reading, writing letters, or watching TV to the early morning, thus severely inhibiting her ability to work with the SS group. But Sara says the rap sessions are especially helpful.

Rose Thomas writes that her support group in Cleveland has been a lifesaver to her, and that members have benefitted from counseling on learning to cope. It all started when several SS patients felt concerned because they could not easily discuss their problems with their families. They did not look ill so it was hard for the families to realize a problem existed. With the encouragement of her doctors and the help of co-worker and friend Joyce Motter, Rose established the Northeast Ohio SS Support Group on February 2, 1987. The only such group in the state, it is attended by thirty-seven members who travel long distances for the meetings. Compassionate doctors from Cleveland hospitals speak about their specialties and the effects of SS. No charges are made for the meetings as it's felt the members already have enough medical expenses to deal with, but free-will offerings are used to mail fliers to hospitals, newspapers, and doctor's offices to help spread the word. "People leave the meetings", Rose says, "with an appreciation for this (support) being opened up to them."

Nurse Jane Tarail is also a writer. When she was diagnosed as having Sjogren's syndrome, she discovered that the nurses she worked with had never heard of her strange illness. Nor had the doctors and dentists she consulted. She decided to write about the syndrome for some medical journals but found them less than enthusiastic. One replied that it couldn't give space to a rare disease no nurse would ever see.

Another indicated it would be interested only if Tarail could furnish them with "hard data - statistics." When the American Journal of Nursing told her to "send the manuscript anyway", she eagerly complied and her article, *Sjogren's Syndrome: A Dry-Eyed Diary* [81] was published in their March 1987 issue. Frustrated by all that disinterest in a malady said to be shared by millions, she decided to locate and band together some of those lonesome sufferers. An ad in a local newspaper turned up eight people from within a thirty-mile-radius and the group was under way. About that time she read in a lupus newsletter about the new Sjogren's Syndrome Foundation (then The Moisture Seekers), and a support group chapter being formed in the area by Audrey Henderson. The two groups joined forces and after some trouble, and with the help of Dr. Troy Daniels, found a meeting place at the University of California at San Francisco. Various health care associations, foundations, hospitals, pharmaceutical corporations, newspapers, and journalists have helped but much of the work of organizing and running the group has fallen on Jane's shoulders, even though she continues to feel that her writing is most important in spreading information about Sjogren's syndrome. Her philosophy, she says, is, "It's a chance to help yourself by helping others, a way to make new friends. By sharing tips, doctor's names, and experiences, you'll have patient power, not patient passivity. SS is a prototype of self-care".

Some support groups have been started by compassionate doctors who see the need to spread information and comfort among their patients. Such a group is the one in Ishikawa, Japan, founded by Dr. Susumu Sugai. Dr. Sugai writes that their first meeting was held in October 1986 and a second in June 1987 at the Kanazawa Medical University Hospital. They were attended by 25 to 30 patients, six physicians, one ophthalmologist, one dentist, a dermatologist, a pharmacologist, three or four nurses and a social worker, and that "a lot of things were spoken of and planned". The latter included a newsletter. Dr. Sugai traces his concern for the patients to the time he spent as a student at the San Francisco clinic. "I stayed in Dr. Talal's laboratory from 1972 to 1974." he says. "I learned a lot of things from him. One day in the late afternoon, he took me to a ward to examine a Sjogren's syndrome patient. On the way to our laboratory he told me a lot of stories of Sjogren's syndrome, saying, 'I love my SS patients.' I was deeply impressed by his words and his attitude toward this disease at that time. I would say that this is the background of starting our SS Association. Secondly, Dr. Shimuzu and I, attending the Copenhagen Symposium, learned how eager the patients were to understand SS. Later I met an SS patient on a boat from Copenhagen to Germany, who told me of the association in the USA. She made me realize how important such an association could be".

In October 1987, Dr. Talal and his research team in San Antonio, Texas, called a meeting of patients to set up a support group there. The doctors spoke of the state of research and their hopes for the future while patients gave the familiar recital of their long paths toward diagnosis before finding their way to the University of Texas clinic. Interested members came from Austin and even as far away as Dallas to form the new SS Foundation chapter. Even at that first enthusiastic meeting, there was talk of breaking off to form separate groups in the two other cities.

These stories are typical of many such groups.

The Arthritis Foundation

An organization which deals with the concerns of all 109 varieties of arthritis (or more properly, connective tissue diseases) is the Arthritis Foundation. Headquartered in Atlanta, Georgia, it supports scientific research, promotes public information and education, and gives direct aid to people in the community who suffer from rheumatic diseases. The Arthritis Foundation co-operates with the American Rheumatism Society, a professional organization of rheumatologists: and The Arthritis Health Professions Association, whose members include nurses, physical and occupational therapists, and medical social workers. Local chapters in many cities conduct seminars and sponsor support groups. A program of self-help courses to aid in coping have been conducted in many cities. The Foundation distributes, free, a series of pamphlets concerning many aspects of arthritis (including one on Sjogren's syndrome) and utilizes in its self-help courses two books, *Arthritis; a Comprehensive Guide* by Dr. James F. Fries, M.D.,[29] Director of the Stanford Arthritis Clinic, and *The Arthritis Helpbook* by Kate Lorig, R.N., Dr. P. H.[46], and Dr. Fries. Although these do not include information specific to Sjogren's syndrome, the two books contain much information that does apply to our problems. In addition the Foundation maintains a list of recommended books on various aspects of arthritis. But more than this, they keep a second list; this one specifies books NOT recommended.

Other publications of the Foundation include their national magazine, *Arthritis Today*, and newsletters published by local chapters. The magazine contains articles by doctors and journalists relating to the business of living with arthritis and even some fiction. There are regular features bringing updates on the state of the world in terms of arthritis. The Foundation provides research fellowships, and helps support research institutions and community centers throughout the country. The local newsletters bring news of seminars and other activities of your local chapter.

Another service provided by the Arthritis Foundation can be particularly helpful for secondary SS patients with debilitating rheumatic disease. The organization's local branches maintain equipment loan closets. They will lend such equipment as wheelchairs at no charge. For patients in search of a doctor, they maintain a list of area rheumatologists. They cannot recommend a specific doctor, but can help you learn which doctors specialize in arthritis diseases and which maintain offices convenient to you.

Prognosis/Support

Other Specific Groups

Another organization that can help Sjogren's syndrome interests is NORD, the National Organization for Rare Disorders. In 1970 a group of national health agencies gathered and found they had a common interest: the fate of patients with diseases so uncommon that they were not profitable for the drug manufacturers. There were therapies that had been developed to help these 'orphans' but the drugs were not being manufactured and so, were not available to the very people who needed them. Some patients were even dying for lack of the only drugs that could help them. Researchers were unable to garner sufficient grant funds to supply their studies. The industry tried to help but the costs of gaining FDA approval were too much for the companies to bear considering the great number of orphan drugs waiting for development. Because of the rarity of the diseases, each organization involved represented too few constituents to have much clout with the FDA, so they joined forces to lobby for congressional action. Jack Klugman, star of television's forensic medicine series *Quincy* learned through his brother Maurice, of their testimony before Congress. In 1981, Klugman broadcast an episode of his popular show dealing with the orphan drug problem. National interest generated by this program nearly swamped the volunteers until NORD was incorporated as a non-profit agency and was able to hire a part time staff. The fledgling organization continued to grow as more and more people made inquiries about rare disorders. A computer database was set up and a networking program now links patients with the same disease with each other and with sources of help. A merger with the National Orphan Drug and Device Foundation, a group set up to fund medical research for rare disorders, allows both organizations to function more efficiently and more effectively. Over 50 agencies (including the Sjogren's Syndrome Foundation) are served by the new agency and countless individual members benefit. In recent years, NORD has been influential in promoting the extension of the Orphan Drug Act and in stimulating the appropriation of funds for research as well as for increasing the awareness of the problem in general. [60] Representatives of the Sjogren's Syndrome Foundation attended the NORD meeting in May 1987 in Washington, D.C. to urge their help in promoting clinical investigations of new medications for SS.

Contact Addresses for Agencies

Sjogren's Syndrome Foundation, Inc.: 29 Gateway Drive, Great Neck, New York 11021 (516) 487-2243

NORD: P. O. Box 8923, New Fairfield, CT 06812 (203) 746-6518

The Arthritis Foundation: 1314 Spring St., N. W., Atlanta, GA 30309 (404) 266-0795

United Scleroderma Foundation: P.O.Box 350, Watsonville, CA 95077 (408) 728-2202

Scleroderma Federation: 1377 K St., NW, Suite 700, Washington, DC 20005 (703) 549-0666

Scleroderma Assoc., Inc.: P.O. Box 910, MA 01940 (617) 334-4910

National Lupus Erythematosus Foundation: 5430 Van Nuys Blvd, Suite 206, Van Nuys CA 91401 (818) 885-8787

Lupus Foundation of America: 11921A Olive Blvd, St Louis, MO 63141 (314) 872-9036

Muscular Dystrophy Association (myositis and dermatomyositis): 810 Seventh Ave., New York NY 10019 (212) 586-0808

Chapter 9

I Think, Therefore I Am

How Your Attitude and Your Doctor's Can Help

It's never easy to hear a doctor tell you you have arthritis. In any form. Rheumatoid arthritis. Scleroderma. Or the one with the impossible name, systemic lupus erythematosis. It takes a while to get chummy enough with that one to shorten it to lupus. Or just SLE. Each separate kind brings with it frightening images of a future filled with pain and disablement. Or worse imagined horrors. The doctor, being kindly, nevertheless, has to say, "We have no cure." You take his prescription, maybe it's just aspirin, and go home feeling very much alone in the world. Chances are you don't know anyone who has arthritis. Oh, Aunt Mabel, maybe, who's all crippled up, but she's old and has always been that way, as long as you can remember. You may be only 35 with a full and busy life that has no room in it for chronic illness. Even the term 'chronic illness' has such a negative tone to it. It's downright depressing. Or it just makes you mad.

You are hesitant to discuss the doctor's verdict with anyone, even your family, at first. Then eventually you find someone, possibly a friend at work, or in the garden club or church, who also has the same sort of aches and pains, although her brand of arthritis may be different than yours. It helps to have someone to share worries with.

It also helps at this particular time to have an understanding and knowledgeable doctor. He'll be willing to take the time to explain your particular situation to you. He'll tell you honestly and frankly, without unduly frightening you, what your prognosis is and how you can help make it better. If he is prescribing medications, he'll explain what they will or will not do for you and what the side effects may be. This can be a difficult proposition for him, as there is almost no chemical that we can put into our bodies that will not have multiple effects. He will tell you where the balance lies with the particular medications you need between risk and important help. He will reassure you. But he will probably wind up saying a lot of it is up to you. You will have to take the medications as he tells you to. You will have to arrange to get the right amount of exercise and rest. But most of all, you will have to adopt a positive attitude. This is far from easy.

Unfortunately, the doctor I have described is not always the one you have to deal with. My files are full of letters from patients who have not had a supportive experience. By far the majority of doctors want to help you adjust but many are busy. Other patients crowd their waiting room, for the time you need. Too often the information you get is just the briefest. And the doctor also has to make a judgement call as to how much to tell you. Sometimes he will feel that too much detail will only make your condition more frightening. This is where the idea of partnership comes in. You must let the doctor know that you want to know, that you want to have an active share in the management of your disease. Give him the guidelines he needs to know how much detail you want to assimilate.

Sjogren's syndrome patients have an additional aspect to the problem. Many of my correspondents tell of years of going from one doctor to another in search of an explanation for a myriad of symptoms. Sadly, the tales are all too often of rebuffs. Of being told they are neurotic. Being told, in essence, to go knit something. Anything to keep you busy and out of the long-suffering doctor's hair. In defense of the beleaguered doctor, I have to say that he is often up against a wall. As we have seen, SS is a very sneaky disease. It masquerades as rheumatoid arthritis, or lupus, or a number of other things. Or you may actually have one of these other diseases. And in that case the symptoms are likely to be readily identifiable and more immediately serious than the SS symptoms. And the SS symptoms are so diverse the doctors often are unable to correlate them.

The hardest part is achieving a balance in all these things. Having a chronic illness is bad enough in itself, but weeping and wailing about it only makes it worse. Henrietta Aladjem, a lupus patient, writes in The Journal of American Medicine[1] that her original diagnosis of lupus was particularly frightening, since at that time, in 1953, the disease was considered rare and invariably fatal. "When I didn't die", she says, "the doctors questioned the diagnosis." It has since been learned that lupus is far less rare and far from being universally fatal, but unfortunately, some patients are still being given that fear. SS and each of its companion diseases carry their own fears and worries. Aladjem points out that alleviating these concerns is not an easy task for the doctor. It takes extra time and a real understanding of the patient's life. There are fears that friends and co-workers will find out about this mysterious ailment and think less of its victim for it, or, conversely, that they will not know, and consider the inevitable fatigue just a case of malingering. The patient may fear being shut out of the mainstream, or being unable to keep pace and compete. He finds it difficult to explain problems to his boss or co-workers as much as to the doctor. As he tries he sees their expressions "change from attentiveness to obvious annoyance". He may even begin to doubt the reality of his own confusing symptoms. It is especially hard then to be sure the doctor does understand. Patient and doctor both find it equally hard to define where the line is between an illness that verges on neurosis, and a neurosis that feeds the illness. Self-doubt, guilt, and a physician who places too much emphasis on the mental aspects of the symptoms can be destructive. My correspondents tell me they have many visits with a psychiatrist before or after their diagnosis. Some say these sessions make them feel better but do little to help the disease. Others swear by the value of the counseling. Rose Thomas, a nursery owner in Chesterland, Ohio, kept a diary of her experiences on the road to diagnosis. In 1982 she experienced blurred vision and difficulty swallowing. Visits to an optometrist and an internist brought tests but little relief. She saw an ophthalmologist in 1983 when a Schirmer test revealed no tears, but no diagnosis was made and artificial tears were suggested. Extreme fatigue in 1984 prompted a regimen of estrogen, but the symptoms continued in 1985. Rose saw eight doctors in 1986 but could not clear up her constant sore throat until February of that year when doctors at University Hospital in Cleveland performed a lip biopsy and gave her the diagnosis of Sjogren's syndrome. They told her it was "incurable, untreatable, not known to go into remission, but livable." By July, the "throat, the eyes, fatigue, pain seemed to be everywhere," and she could not cope. She was referred to a clinical psychiatrist whose suggestions consisted of relaxation through breathing exercises along with instructions for living one day at a time. Rose finds this very effective and says she highly recommends counseling. She also reports that the support group is extremely valuable and she includes prayer in her regular routine.

Positive Thinking

All this indicates that, though we all know that SS is certainly not "all in the mind", a patient's mental attitude makes a tremendous difference in her ability to manage her Sjogren's and to live a full and rewarding life. Studies by husband-and-wife team Janice Kiecott-Glaser and Ronald Glaser of Ohio State University indicated that men and women involved in divorces or unhappy marriages had weakened immune systems and lowered ability to fight off infections. But, in a possible explanation of the comfort found in sharing experiences with members of the SS support groups, another study, concluded that talking about emotional problems actually strengthened a person's immune responses.[11] This study was reported to the American Psychological Association's 1987 meeting by Southern Methodist University's Jamie Pennebaker.

Achieving a healthful mental state is not easy with Sjogren's syndrome, but it can and must be done. Your doctor, friends, family, and fellow sufferers can all help, but ultimately it is your own outlook and approach to life that will make the difference, and minimize that second problem that comes with the territory. If we can't get rid of the syndrome, at least we can learn to live with it.

Glossary

GLOSSARY OF TERMS RELATED TO SJOGREN'S SYNDROME

Achlorhydria - lack of hydrochloric acid in gastric juice

Acupressure - compression of blood vessels by means of needles

Acupuncture - technique for treating pain by inserting needles into specific parts of the body

Adenopathy - swelling of lymph nodes

Adrenal glands - Supply hormones such as cortisone, estrogen, progesterone, and androgen

Alzheimer's Disease - Progressive brain disease characterized by premature deterioration of intellectual function

ANA - Antinuclear antibody, a marker for lupus

Androgen - Male hormone

Antigen - substance that when introduced into the body stimulates the production of an antibody

Anti-La antibody - found in serum of primary SS patients

Anti-Ro antibody - found in serum of primary SS patients

Antibody - protein substance developed by the body to counteract a specific antigen

Arthritis Foundation - Support organization for arthritis patients

Artificial tears - drops designed to replace natural tears

Autoimmune disease - disorder in which the body's immune system reacts against healthy tissue

B cells - Lymphocyte (white blood cell) formed in bone marrow to produce antibodies

Biopsy - removal of a small piece of tissue to be studied microscopically

Bone marrow - soft organic material filling bone cavities

Break up time (BUT) - Test to measure quality of tear film on eye

Bromhexine - Experimental drug to increase production of saliva, tears, and bronchial secretions
Bronchitis - inflammation of mucous membranes of the bronchial tubes
Candidiasis - a form of yeast infection attacking skin or mucous membranes
Cellular immunity - the mechanical process of warding off foreign substances by white cells
Chyme - ball of semi-digested food as it progresses through stomach and intestines
Cirrhosis - a chronic, degenerative disease of the liver
Conjunctivitis - inflammation of the mucous membrane lining the eyelids
Connective tissue - supports and connects other tissues and body parts
Connective tissue disease - disorders characterized by inflammation of connective tissues and blood vessels (includes SLE, scleroderma, polymyositis, dermatomyositis, and polyarteritis)
Corticosteroid - hormones produced by the adrenal glands
Cricoid cartilage - ring-like cartilage at lower part of larynx
Cytotoxic drugs - chemicals that destroy cells, used as cancer fighting drugs when specific for fast growing cells
Dermatomyositis - chronic disease characterized by fluid retention, skin irritations, weakness and inflammation of the muscles
Diverticulitis - inflammation of sacs in the lining of the intestines and colon
Dysphagia - difficulty in swallowing
Dyspnea - difficulty in breathing
Efamol - trade name for oil of evening primrose, experimentally used in treatment of SS
Electron microscope - utilizes a stream of electrons for greatly magnified images of objects
Enzymes - proteins that induce chemical changes in other substances without being changed themselves, i.e.; in digestive juices they are

Glossary

capable of breaking down foods into compounds usable by the body
Epistaxis - nosebleed
Epithelial cells - form the outer layer of the body and the linings of cavities
Erythrocyte - mature red blood cell
Erythema - red color in inflamed area
Esophagus - muscular tube carrying food from pharynx to stomach
Estrogen - female sex hormone
Etiology - causes of disease
Eustachian tube - leads from middle ear to pharynx, lined with mucous membrane
Evening primrose oil - see Efamol
Exocrine gland - glands whose secretions reach and lubricate the skin or mucous membranes
Fatty acid - acids important to the digestive process
Filamentary keratitis - inflammation of the cornea with stringy strands of epithelial cells
Fluorescein dye - used in testing for damage to cornea
Fluoride - a compound applied topically to teeth for prevention of decay
Gamma-linolenic acid - a fatty acid
Gastric glands - tubular glands in the mucous lining of the stomach
Goiter - an enlargement of the thyroid gland
Gold salts - injections used in treatment of rheumatoid arthritis or lupus
Gougerot's syndrome - a general condition in which the eyes, mouth, larynx, nose, and vulva all suffered from a related dryness which also affected the thyroid and ovaries (described by French physician Dr. H. Gougerot)
Gynecologist - a specialist in diseases of the female reproductive system
Helper T cells - lymphocytes designed to alert the immune system
Hepatitis - a disorder characterized by inflammation of the liver
HLA - human leukocyte antigen

Humoral immunity - chemical immune action initiated by B cells producing antibodies in the blood serum
Hydrochloric acid - a normal constituent of digestive juice
Hypotonic - a solution of lower osmotic pressure than another
IgA - an immunoglobulin
Immune system - organs of the body involved in producing immune reactions
Immune tolerance - the ability of an immune cell to know when NOT to react violently to another substance
Immunoglobulins - proteins capable of acting as antibodies
Immunosuppressive drugs - substances that interfere with the normal immune response. Used to protect foreign tissue grafts and in combatting autoimmune diseases
Indocin - a non-steroidal anti-inflammatory drug
Internist - a specialist in diseases of the internal organs
Interstitial cystitis - inflammation of the lining of the bladder
Interstitial nephritis - inflammation of connective tissue of kidneys
Keratoconjunctivitis sicca (KCS) - a condition of dry eyes caused by lymphocytic infiltration of the tear glands
Killer T cells - lymphocytes which destroy invading foreign substances
Lacrimal glands - secrete tears to lubricate the eyes
Lactoferrin - protein found in tears and saliva
Lagothpthalmos, nocturnal - incomplete closure of the eyelids during sleep
Larynx - Upper end of the throat, a cartilage structure lined with mucous membrane, "voice box"
Liver - organ which secretes bile and contributes to metabolic functions; is main site for production of plasma proteins

Glossary

Lupus Foundation of America - Support organization for lupus patients

Lymphocytes - White blood cells forming "soldiers" of the immune system

Lymphoma - malignant growth of cells in lymph system

Marker - gene or trait that identifies linked traits

Mixed connective tissue disease (MCTD) - a combination of four different disorders

Meibomian glands - tear glands in the eyelids

Mikulicz' disease - disorder described by Dr. Johann von Mikulicz-Radecki involving sicca syndrome. Later determined to be identical to Sjogren's syndrome.

Mucolytic agent - drops to dissolve excess mucus

Mucous membranes - lining of passages and cavities communicating with the air, usually containing mucus secreting glands

Mucus - thick fluid secreted by mucous membranes and glands

National Lupus Erythematosus Foundation - support organization for lupus patients

National Organization for Rare Diseases (NORD) - Support organization for a variety of 'orphan' diseases

Natural killer (NK) cells - white cells programed to destroy 'invaders'

Neonatal lupus erythematosus (NLE) - Lupus-like symptoms seen in infants born to women with SS markers

Nodule - small aggregation of cells sometimes seen under the skin in immune system disorders, also normal structural unit of lymph tissue

Non-steroidal anti-inflammatory drug (NSAID) - group of drugs used to treat inflammatory disorders

Osmotic pressure - tension between two solutions of different concentrations separated by a semipermeable membrane

Otitis - inflammation of the ear

Pancreas - digestive system gland that produces insulin for the metabolism of carbohydrates plus digestive pancreatic juice
Pancreatitis - inflammation of the pancreas
Parkinson's disease - chronic nervous disorder characterized by tremor, muscular weakness, and rigidity caused by a deficiency in the brain's production of the chemical dopamine
Parotid gland - major salivary gland
Penicillamine - derivative of penicillin used in treatment of rheumatoid arthritis
Phagocytes - white cell that destroys foreign particles by literally 'eating' them
Pharynx - passageway for air from nasal cavity to larynx and for food from mouth to esophagus
Philocarpine - experimental drug used to stimulate saliva production.
Photosensitivity - over reaction to light
Plaque - gummy mass of micro-organisms that grows on teeth and promotes decay
Pleurisy - inflammation of the membrane that encloses the lungs
Pneumonia - inflammation of the lungs
Polyarteritis - inflammation of the medium and small arteries
Polymyositis - disorder of the connective tissue characterized by inflammation and degeneration of the muscles
Prednisone - a steroid hormone produced by the adrenal glands
Primary Sjogren's syndrome - sicca complex symptoms without underlying connective tissue disease
Prostaglandins - fatty acid derivatives present in and affecting many issues including the brain, lung, kidney, thymus, and pancreas
Psuedo-lymphoma - clusters of non-malignant cells giving the false appearance of true lymphomas
Puncta - ducts for drainage of excess tears into nasal cavity

Glossary

Punctal occlusion - procedure to block puncta, retaining tears in eye

Purpura - red to purple areas under the skin caused by hemorrhages of small blood vessels usually found on the legs in SS or in sun-exposed areas when a side effect of corticosteroid treatment

Raynaud's phenomenon - condition where the fingers become very sensitive to cold, heat, or emotional stress

Rheumatoid arthritis (RA) - Autoimmune disorder characterized by inflammation of the joints

Rheumatoid factor - immunoglobulin present in serum of 50 to 95% of adults with rheumatoid arthritis

Rheumatologist - specialist in rheumatic diseases

Rhinitis - inflammation of the nasal lining

Rose-bengal dye - used to detect effects of dry eye damage

Salicylates - Aspirin-like drugs

Saline - salty

Salivary ducts - tubes connecting salivary glands to mouth

Salivary glands - glands which secrete fluids to lubricate and protect mouth

Schirmer test - used to measure secretion of tears

Scintiscan - method of measuring fluids utilizing radioactive substances

Scleroderma - chronic connective tissue disease characterized by irritation of the skin and organs of the gastrointestinal tract, lungs, heart, and kidneys

Scleroderma Federation - support organization for scleroderma patients

Secondary Sjogren's syndrome - sicca symptoms experienced in combination with an underlying connective tissue disease

Sed rate (erythrocyte sedimentation rate) - test of the speed at which erythrocytes settle in the blood, used to indicate presence of inflammatory disease

Sialogram - record of examination of salivary glands with x-rays

Sicca complex - related symptoms of dry eyes and dry mouth
Sjogren's Syndrome Foundation (SSF) - support organization for SS patients
Sjogren's syndrome (SS) - a chronic systemic autoimmune disorder characterized by dry eys and dry mouth (sicca complex) with joint pain
Slit lamp - lamp constructed so that an intense light is emitted through a slit for the examination of the eye
Spleen - capsule of lymph tissue engaged in the production and storage of blood cells and blood filtration
SS-A, SS-B - genetic markers for Sjogren's syndrome
Steroids - hormones produced in the adrenal glands
Sublingual glands - salivary glands found under the tongue
Submaxillary glands - salivary glands found in the floor of the mouth
Suppressor T cells - lymphocytes geared to inhibit the action of killer cells
Synovial capsule - enclosure formed by synovial membrane around joint
Synovial membrane - membrane enclosing the lubricating fluid of a joint
Synovitis - inflammation of the synovial membrane
Systemic - pertaining to the whole body, rather than one of its parts
Systemic lupus erythematosus (SLE) - chronic inflammatory connective tissue disorder affecting the skin, joints, kidneys, nervous system, and mucous membranes
T cells - lymphocytes (white blood cells) developed in the thymus programmed to alert immune system, destroy invading foreign cells, and suppress antibody-forming action of B cells
Trans mandibular joint (TMJ) - joint connecting lower jaw to skull
United Scleroderma Foundation - support organization for scleroderma patients
Vaginitis - inflammation of the vagina

Glossary

Van Bijsterveld score - dry-eye measure using rose-bengal staining
Vasculitis - inflammation of the blood vessels
Vitreous body - jelly-like substance filling the cavity of the eyeball
Waldenstrom's macroglobulinemia - disorder characterized by excessive production of immunoglobulins causing anemia, lassitude, confusion, and bleeding
Xerophthalmia - dry eye condition caused by vitamin A deficiency
Xerostomia - dry mouth caused by lack of saliva

Bibliography

1. Aladjem, H. Psychosocial aspects of Rheumatic Disease - a Patient Speaks - A Primer on Rheumatic Diseases. Journal of American Medical Associalion; 1973; 224: 205-206.

2. Alarcon-Segovia D. Symptomatic Sjogren's Syndrome in Mixed Connective Tissue Disease. The Journal of Rheumatology; 1984; 11: 582-583.

3. Alexander, E. Inflammatory Vascular Disease in Sjogren's Syndrome. Sjogren's Syndrome, Clinical and Immunological Aspects. Berlin: Springer-Verlag; August, 1987.

4. Alexander, E. Neuromuscular Complications of Primary Sjogren's Syndrome. Sjogren's Syndrome, Clinical and Immunological Aspects. Berlin: Springer-Verlag; August, 1987.

5. Alexander, E. The Relationship Between Anti-RO (SS-A) Precipitin Antibody Positive Sjogren's Syndrome and Anti-RO (SS-A) Precipitin Antibody Positive Lupus Erythematosus. Sjogren's Syndrome, Clinical and Immunological Aspects. Berlin: Springer-Verlag; August, 1987.

6. Alexander E. et al . Primary Sjogren's Syndrome with Central Nervous System Disease Mimicking Multiple Sclerosis. Annals of Internal Medicine; 1986; 104: 323-330.

7. Alexander M. Clinical Aspects of Sjogren's Syndrome. Southern Medical Journal; July 1986; 79: 857-862.

8. American Academy of Ophthalmology. Dry Eye/Understanding your condition: Pamphlet; 1985.

9. American Academy of Ophthalmology. Floaters and Flashers: Pamphlet; 1985.

10. Anderson L., Talal N. The Spectrum of Benign to Malignant Lymphoproliferation in Sjogren's Syndrome. Clinical Experimental Immunology; 1971; 9: 199-221.

11. AP/New York. Immune Systems Linked to Marriage, Houston Post; 29 August, 1987.

12. Arnett F. HLA Genes and Predisposition to Rheumatic Diseases. Hospital Practice; 1986: 89-100.

13. Arthritis Foundation. Polymyositis and Dermatomyositis. Atlanta, GA: AF; 1985.

14. Arthritis Foundation. Rheumatoid Arthritis. Atlanta, GA: AF; 1983.

15. Arthritis Foundation. Scleroderma. Atlanta, GA: AF; 1983.

16. Arthritis Foundation. Sjogren's Syndrome. Atlanta, GA: AF; 1985.

17. Arthritis Foundation. Systemic Lupus Erythematosus. Atlanta, GA: AF; 1984.

18. Bariffi F. et al. Pulmonary Involvement in Sjogren's Syndrome. Respiration ; 1984; 46: 82-87.

19. Booth, A. B. Walking For Arthritis. Arthritis Today; October 1987: 10-12.

20. Chudwin et al. Spectrum of Sjogren's Syndrome in Children. The Journal of Pediatrics; February 1981; 98: 312-217.

21. Constantopoulos S. et al. Respiratory Manifestations in Primary Sjogren's Syndrome. Ionnina, Greece: University of Ionnina.

Bibliography

22. Constantopoulos S. et al. Xerotrachea and Interstitial Lung Disease in Primary Sjogren's Syndrome. Respiration; 1984; 46: 310-314.

23. Daniels T. et al . Sjogren's Syndrome Clinic, University of CA/San Francisco; May, 1985.

24. DeLuise, V., Peterson, W. The Use of Topical Healon ™ Tears in the Management of Refractory Dry-eye Syndrome. Annals of Ophthalmology; September 1984: 823-824.

25. Drosos, A et al. Cyclosporin A Therapy in Patients with Primary Sjogren's Syndrome: Results at One Year. Scandinavian Journal of Rheumatology; 1986; Suppl. 61: 246-249.

26. Dustman, R. Brisk Walk Aids Mind, Studies Say. UPI,Chicago: Houston Post; 30 August 1987.

27. Editors of Consumer Reports Books. Consumer's Union's Peport on False Health Claims, Worthless Remedies, and Unproved Therapies. Mount Vernon, New York: Consumers Union; 1980.

28. Fox, R. et al. First International Symposium on Sjogren's Syndrome: Suggested Criteria for Classification. Scandinavian Journal of Rheumatology; 1986; Suppl. 61: 28-30.

29. Fries, J. Arthritis. A Comprehensive Guide. Reading, Massachusetts: Addison-Wesley Publishing Company; 1979.

30. Gumpel, J. Sjogren's Syndrome. British Medical Journal; 4 December 1982; 285: 6355, 1598.

31. Harris, E. Editor. Boehringer to undertake Development of Bisolvon as SS Medication. The Moisture Seekers, Great Neck, NY; February 1988; 5: 1.

32. Harris, E. The SSF - 1983, Today, and Our Future. The Moisture Seekers, Great Neck, NY; July-Aug, 1987; 4: 7, 1.

33. Henkin, R. I. et al. Abnormalities of Taste and Smell in Sjogren's Syndrome . Annals of Internal Medicine; 1972; 76: 375-383.

34. Homma, M. et al. Criteria for Sjogren's Syndrome in Japan. Scandinavian Journal of Rheumatology; 1986; Suppl. 61: 26-27.

35. Ichikawa Y, et al. Circulating Natural Killer Cells in Sjogren's Syndrome. Arthritis and Rheumatism; Feb 1985; 28: 182-187.

36. Jabs, D. et al. Familial Abnormalities of Lymphocyte Function in a Large Sjogren's Syndrome Kindred. The Journal of Rheumatology; 1986; 13: 320-326.

37. Jameson E. The Natural History of Quackery. Springfield IL: Charles C Thomas, Publishers; 1961.

38. Kaltreider, H. et al. The Neuropathy of Sjogren's Syndrome. Annals of Internal Medicine; April 1969; 70: 751-761.

39. Katz, S. G-I Problems Associated With SS. The Moisture Seekers Newsletter, Great neck, NY; October, 1987; 4: 1.

40. Kaufman, H. Keratitis Sicca. International Ophthalmological Clinic; Summer 1984; 24: 133-43.

41. Kjellen, G. et al. Esophageal Function, Radiography, and Dysphagia in Sjogren's Syndrome. Digestive Diseases and Sciences; March 1986; 31: 225-229.

42. Koffler, D. The Immunology of Rheumatoid Diseases. Clinical Symposia; 1979; 37.

Bibliography

43. Konttinen, Yrio T. et al. Lactoferrin in Sjogren's Syndrome. Arthritis and Rheumatism; April 1984; 27: 462-466.

44. Lang, P. . Dr. Paul Lang, Allergist, Addresses November Meeting. Moisture Seekers Newsletter, Great Neck, NY; December, 1986; 3: 11.

45. Leonardo, E. et al. Autoimmune Aspects in a Case of Chronic Interstitial Cystitis. Minerva Medica; June 1986; 77.

46. Lorig, K., Fries, J. The Arthritis Helpbook. Reading, Massachusetts: Addison-Wesley Publishing Company; 1980.

47. Malinow, K. et al . Neuropsychiatric Dysfunction in Primary Sjogren's Syndrome. Annals of Internal Medicine; 1985; 103: 344-349.

48. Manthorpe, R. et al. The Copenhagen Criteria for Sjogren's Syndrome. Scandinavian Journal of Rheumatology; 1986; Suppl. 61: 19-21.

49. Manthorpe, R. et al. Editorial Comments to the Four Sets of Criteria for Sjogren's Syndrome. Scandinavian Journal of Rheumatology; 1986; Suppl. 61: 31-35.

50. Manthorpe, R., Prause, J. Message of Welcome. Scandinavian Journal of Rheumatology; 1986; Suppl. 61: 11.

51. Manthorpe,R, Prause, J. Treatment of Sjogren's Syndrome: An Overview. Scandinavian Journal of Rheumatology; 1986; Suppl. 61: 237.

52. Manthorpe R. et al. Sjogren's Syndrome: A Review with Emphasis on Immunological Features. Allergy; 1981; 36: 139-153.

53. Michelson, P. (Scripps Clinic, La Jolla CA). Living With Dry Eyes.

54. Mizel, S., Jaret, P. In Self Defense. New York: Harcourt Brace Jovanovich, Publishers; 1985.

55. Molina, R. et al. Primary Sjogren's Syndrome in Men. The American Journal of Medicine; Jan 1980; 80: 23-31.

56. Molina, R. Rudy Molina Discusses Vasculitis at Greater Washington Meeting. Great Neck, NY; January 1987; 4: 1-3.

57. Morgan, W., Castleman, B. A Clinicopathologic Study of "Mikulicz's Disease". American Journal of Pathology; 1953; 29: 471.

58. Moutsopoulos, H. et al. Differences in the Clinical Manifestations of Sicca Syndrome in the Presence and Absence of Rheumatoid Arthritis. The American Journal of Medicine; May 1979; 66: 733-736.

59. National Institute of Dental Research. Dry Mouth (Xerostomia). Bethesda, MD: Pamphlet.

60. Nord. What is NORD. NORD Newsletter, New Fairfield, CN; 5: 1.

61. Oldstone, M. AP/NewYork (from Science). Viruses May Be Good for You. Palm Beach Post; 1 February 1988.

62. Papathanasiou, M. et al. Reappraisal of Respiratory Abnormalities in Primary and Secondary Sjogren's Syndrome. Chest; September 1986; 90: 370-374.

63. Pavlidis, N. et al. The Clinical Picture of Primary Sjogren's Syndrome: a Retrospective Study. Journal of Rheumatology; 1982; 9: 685-689.

Bibliography

64. Reveille, J. et al. Primary Sjogren's Syndrome and Other Autoimmune Diseases in Families. Annals of Internal Medicine; 1984; 101: 748-756.

65. Rooney, E., Lindsley, H. Sjogren's Syndrome - An Update. The Journal of the Kansas Medical Society; September 1983: 482-485.

66. Ruiz-Arguelles, G. The "Lipstick-on-Teeth" Sign in Sjogren's Syndrome. New England Journal of Medicine; Oct. 16, 1986; 315: 16.

67. Sciubba, J. et al, Moderator. Report on September 86 Symposium: Living with Sjogren's III, Part 2. Moisture Seekers Newsletter, Great Neck, NY; March 1987; 4: 1-5.

68. Sciubba, J.,Borgia, L., Speaker NYC Meeting. Untitled report. Moisture Seekers, Great Neck. NY; June, 1987; 4: 6, 1-5.

69. Segerberg-Konttinen, M. et al. Focus Score in the Diagnosis of Sjogren's Syndrome. Scandinavian Journal of Rheumatology; 1986; Suppl. 61: 47-51.

70. Shearn, M. Sjogren's Syndrome. Philadelphia: W. B. Saunders; 1971.

71. Sheehy, T. . Dr. Thomas Sheehy, Jr. Discusses Gynecological Problems Related to Sjogren's Syndrome. Moisture Seekers Newsletter, Great Neck, NY; May, 1986; 3: 5, 1-7.

72. Skopouli, F. et al. Preliminary Diagnostic Criteria for Sjogren's Syndrome. Scandinavian Journal of Rheumatology; 1986; Suppl. 61: 22-25.

73. Strimlan, C. Pulmonary Involvement in Sjogren's Syndrome. Chest; June 1986; 89: 901-902.

74. Talal, N. Curriculum Vitae; May 8 1987.

75. Talal, N. How to Recognise and Treat Sjogren's Syndrome. Drug Therapy ; June 1984: 80-87.

76. Talal, N. Ahmed, A. Immunoregulation by Hormones - An Area of Growing Importance. The Journal of Rheumatology; 1987; 14: 191-193.

77. Talal, N., Smith, L. Recent Clinical and Experimental Developments in Sjogren's Syndrome. Western Journal of Medicine; January, 1975; 122: 50-58.

78. Talal, N. Sex Hormones and Modulation of Immune Response in SLE. Clinics in Rheumatic Diseases; April 1982; 8: 23-27.

79. Talal, N. Sjogren's Syndrome and Connective Tissue Disease with other Immunological Disorders. McCarty. Arthritis and Related Conditions. Philadelphia: Lea & Febiger; 1985-87.

80. Talal, N, Editor. Sjogren's Syndrome, Clinical and Immunological Aspects. Berlin: Springer-Verlag; August, 1987.

81. Tarail, J.,Teutsch, E. Sjogren's Syndrome: a Dry-Eyed Diary/Adding Moisture to Your Life. American Journal of Nursing
; March, 1987: 324-329.

82. Thomas C. Taber's Cyclopedic Medical Dictionary. Philadelphia: F. A. Davis Company; 1985.

83. Torinto, S. et al. Dictionary of Medical Syndromes: Sjogren's I. Philadelphia: J. B. Lippincott Co.; 1921; 750.

Bibliography

84. Tseng,S. (Massachusetts Eye and Ear Infirmary, Harvard Medical School). Topical Vitamin A Treatment for Dry Eye Disorders. Washington, DC: Research to Prevent Blindness, Inc.; 2 Oct. 1984; Science Writers Semminar in Ophthalmology.

85. Udell, I. Dry Eye (Keratitis Sicca). Carsons, S. Sjogren's Syndrome: Distinguishing Primary From Secondary. Great Neck, NY: SSFoundation; March 10, 1987.

86. UT Health Science Center. Rheumatology/Clinical Immunology Fellowship Training,Dept of Medicine, UT Health Science Center at San Antonio; Brochure; 1987.

87. Van Mulders, A. et al. Hypergastrinemia in Rheumatoid Arthritis Related to Sjogren's Syndrome. The Journal of Rheumatology; 1984; 11: 246.

88. Watson, R. et al. Neonatal Lupus Erythematosus: A Clinical Seriological and Immunogenetic Study with Review of Literature. Medicine; 1984; 63: 362-378.

89. Whelton, J et al. Heberden's Nodes, Dip Erosions and Systemic Findings. Washington DC; 220.

90. Witter, D. C.; Dickey, P. H. Relaxation: A Treat of a Treatment for Pain. Arthritis Today; October 1987: 28-31.

91. Woldheim, F. Henrik Sjogren and Sjogren's Syndrome. Scandinavian Journal of Rheumatology; 1986; Suppl: 61: 12-15.

92. Wright, W. Oral Health Care Program Recommended by National Institute of Dental Research of NIH. Moisture Seekers Newsletter, Great Neck, NY; January, 1987; 4: 1, 1-2.

Index

INDEX

Abdominal pain 29
Abelson, Dr. Mark 115
Achalasia 30
Achlorhydria 30
Acid secreting glands 28, 29, 30
Acidity 30, 50, 84
Acupressure 98
Acupuncture 98
Adhatoda vasica, 109
Adrenal glands 84, 85
Aging 105
Ahmed, Dr. S. Ansar 49, 108
Air conditioning 25, 116
Aladjem, Henrietta 125
Alexander, Dr. Elaine L. 37, 105
Alkalinity 50
Allergy 35, 63, 114
American Academy of Ophthalmology 19
American Association of Pathologists and Bacteriologists 59
American Journal of Medicine 104
American Journal of Nursing 118
American Psychological Association 127
American Rheumatism Association 60, 104
American Rheumatism Society 119
Amino acids 50
Androgens 108
Anemia 71
Angina 30

Ankles 23, 37
Antibodies 45, 46, 51 53, 71, 108, 112
Antidepressants 68
Antidiuretic hormones 28
Antihigh blood pressure drugs 68
Antihistamines 34, 68
Anti-inflammatory drugs 28
Anti-La (SS-B) antibody 51, 69
Antinuclear antibodies (ANA) 53, 71
Anti-Ro (SS-A) antibody 51, 69, 105
Antigens 46, 47, 53
Appetite 37
Arnett, Dr. Frank 9, 37, 105, 110
Arthritis 32, 57-59, 60, 77, 82, 84, 88, 93, 97, 98, 107, 119
Arthritis, A Comprehensive Guide 98, 119
Arthritis and Allied Conditions 104
Arthritis Foundation Clinical Center 104
Arthritis Foundation, Inc. 88, 89, 116, 119-120, 122
Arthritis Health Professions Association 119
Arthritis Helpbook, The 70, 119
Arthritis Today 93, 119
Artificial tears 73, 75, 77

Aspirin 28, 82, 98
Audie L. Murphy Veterans Administration Hospital 103
Auto-antibodies 68
Autoimmunity 11, 47-49, 52, 63, 65, 104, 108, 109
B cells 45
Bacteria 20, 46, 50
Bartholin's glands 26, 97
Bee sting venom 98
Bicarbonate 50
Bile acids 84
Billruth, Dr. Christian A. T. 56
Biopsy 63, 68, 69, 71
Bisolvon™ 109
Bladder problems 28
Blood cells 16, 34, 87
Blood serum 32, 46, 77
Blood tests 64, 68, 69, 71, 87
Blood vessels 18, 26, 27, 37
Blurred vision 126
Boehringer-Ingelheim Pharmaceuticals Inc 109
Bone marrow 44
Breakup time (BUT) 64, 67
British Medical Journal 65
Bromhexide hydrochloride 77
Bromhexine 109
Bronchitis 24, 109
Burning sensation 25, 27, 30
Calcium 20, 50, 85, 88, 95
California Criteria 52-64, 65
Cancer 68, 81, 86, 97
Candidiasis 21

Carpal tunnel syndrome 31
Carsons, Dr. Steven 115
Cartilage 87
Cataracts 85
Cavities 20
Cellular immunity 46
Central nervous system 27, 31
Chemotherapy 47, 61, 68, 81
Chest pain 24, 30
Chest xrays 70, 71
Chewing gum 19
Chloride 50
Choking 21, 29
Cholesterol 84
Chyme 29
Cirrhosis 30
Clinical Immunology and Arthritis Section 103
Cod liver oil 98
Columbia University 104
Congenital defects 47
Congested ears 35
Congestion 24, 25, 35
Connective tissue cells 59
Connective tissue disease 7, 8, 10, 11, 13, 36, 38, 64, 70, 73, 88, 90, 107
Constantopoulos 106
Constipation 29
Consumers' Union 101
Contact lenses 18, 76
Copenhagen Criteria 62, 64
Copenhagen Symposium 62, 64, 119
Copper bracelet 97
Cornea, clouding (opacity) 18

Index

Corneal abrasion 18, 77
Corneal ulcers 112
Corticosteroids 81
Cortisone 84
Criteria for diagnosis 62
Cyclosporin A 110
Cytotoxic drugs 81
Danazol 108
Daniels, Dr. Troy 104, 105, 115, 118
deLuise, Dr. Vincent 115
Depression 26, 31, 37, 85
Dermatomyositis 7, 10, 13, 36, 38, 88, 122
Diagnosis 60, 61-71, 106, 107, 110, 126
Diamond, Dr. Herbert S. 115
Diarrhea 29
Dickey, Pat Hamilton 93
Diet 19, 21, 29
Difficulties in concentration 31
Digestive system 21, 24-29, 30, 38, 82, 95, 96
Diverticulitis 29
Division of Clinical Immunology and Arthritis (UTSA) 103
Dizziness 84
DMSO 98
Drug Therapy 12
Dry cough 24
Dry eyes 1, 10, 15-19, 31, 57, 61, 63, 64, 65, 73-77, 105, 115
Dry hair 27
Dry mouth 1, 5, 10, 15, 16, 19-22, 24, 27, 50, 57, 59, 65, 77-81, 114
Dry scalp 27

Dry skin 2, 24, 84, 94-95
Dry throat 21-22
Duodenum 29
Dustman, Dr. Robert 90
Efamol (Evening primrose oil) 109
Elbows 37
Electrocardiogram 71
Electrolytes 28
Electron microscopes 44
Emotional upset 18, 26
Endorphins 89
Endress, Sara 21, 25, 80, 116-117
Enemas 98
Enzymes 21, 29, 50
Esophagus 21, 24, 30, 71, 96
Estrogen 108, 126
Eustachian tubes 25
Exercise 73, 87-92, 126
Exocrine glands 10, 11, 24, 63, 111
Extra-glandular Symptoms 27, 28, 70, 112
Eye Clinic at Heidelberg Congress 55
Eyes *see Dry eyes*
Farris, Dr. R. Linsy 115
Fatigue 5, 35, 37, 116
Fatty acid 109
Fever 38
Fifth rash, the 4
Filamentary Keratitis 56
Fingers 27, 31, 38, 53
Flashes, floaters, and zig-zags 18, 19
Fluorescein dye 65
Flu shots 98
Fluoride 20, 80
Flushing 85

Focus score 68
Food and Drug Administration (FDA) 109, 121
Fox, Dr. Philip 105, 109
Fries, Dr. James F. 93, 98, 101, 120
Frequent urination 27, 53
Functioning fluid 46
Fungus 50
Furie, Dr. Richard 115
Gamma-Linolenic Acid 109
Gas 29
Gastric glands 29
Genes 47, 51, 52, 53
Gilbard, Dr. Jeffrey 115
Glaser 127
Goblet cells 110
Goiter 52
Gold salts 86
Gougerot's syndrome 57
Greenspan, Dr. John 115
Greenwald, Dr. Robert A. 115
Greek Criteria 62-64
Groin 34
Gumpel, J. M. 65
Hadden, Dr. W. B. 57
Hands 37
Harris, Elaine 114, 116
Harvard Medical School 110
Hashimoto's thyroiditis 60
Heart blockage 36, 112
Healon 78
Heartburn 30, 96
Hench, Dr. Philip S. 84
Henderson, Audrey 118
Hepatitis 47
High fibre foods 29

Hips 87, 89, 90
Histamine 34
HLA complexes 36, 51, 52, 53
Hoarseness 24
Holland 106
Holm, Dr. S. 59
Hormones 28, 49, 84, 85
Humidifiers 76
Humoral immunity 46
Hyaluronic acid 78
Hydrochloric acid 29, 96
Hygiea 58
Hyperglobulinemia 60
Hypochondria 114
Hypotonic 75
Immune system 10, 34, 37, 38, 43-54, 86, 107-109, 129
Immune tolerance 47
Immunoglobulins 34, 35, 45, 46, 50
Immunosuppressive drugs 84, 86
Indigestion 29
Inflammation 19, 22, 23, 25, 26, 28, 30, 31, 37, 38, 64, 68, 70, 84, 85, 87, 89, 90, 94, 96
Institut de Recherches Scientifiques sur le Cancer in Paris 104
Institute of Eye Pathology, Copenhagen 62
International Ophthalmological Clinic 75
Interstitial cystitis 28, 98
Intestinal problems 28, 29

Index

Investigational New Drug 109
Iron deposits 85
Itching 35
Jacobson, Dr. Edmund 93
Jabs, Dr. Douglas 105
Jameson, Eric 99
Japanese Criteria 62, 64
Japanese Health and Welfare Ministry 105
Johns Hopkins University 105
Joints 1, 2, 3, 4, 8, 10, 11, 15, 23, 36, 37, 38, 52, 53, 61, 63, 67, 82, 84, 87, 100, 101
Journal of American Medicine 125
Kalweit 56
Kanazawa Medical University Hospital 118
Kapalin, Bernice 17, 26, 112
Karolinska Institute 57
Karsh, Dr. 107
Kassan, Dr. Robert J. v
Kassan, Dr. S. S. 103
Katz, Dr. Seymour 30, 95
Kaufman, Dr. Herbert 76
Keratoconjunctivitis sicca (KCS) 12, 16-19, 55, 56, 57, 58, 63, 64, *see Dry eyes*
Kerpen, Dr. Howard 109
Kidneys 27, 28, 37, 38, 70, 87
Kiecott-Glaser, Janice 127
Klugman, Jack 121
Klugman, Maurice 121
Knees 37, 87, 90
Knuckles 89

Lacrimal glands 17
Lactoferrin 50
Lactose intolerance 95
Lane, Dr. H. Clifford 116
Lang, Dr. Paul 114
Larynx 24, 30, 60
Leber, Dr. 55
Linings of the heart 37
Lipstick smears 20
Liver 27, 30
Long Island Jewish Medical Center 30, 109
Lorig, Kate 93, 120
Loss of fat cells 26
Loss of hearing sharpness 25
Lower respiratory system 24
Lubricating sheath 23
Lull, Aileen 23
Lump in your throat 21
Lund University 107
Lungs 24, 37, 38, 106
Lupus 7, 9, 13, 35, 36, 37, 48, 52, 53, 69, 71, 105, 108, 112, 118, 122
Lupus Foundation of America 122
Lymphocytes 11, 17, 19, 28, 31, 32, 43-54, 63, 64, 65, 68, 86, 105, 108, 110
Lymphoma 32, 107
Lymph node 34, 107
Mandel, Dr. Irwin 116
Manthorpe, Dr. Rolf 62, 107, 109
Massachusetts Eye and Ear Infirmary 110
Mast cells 34
McCarty, D. J. 104

Medical Advisory Board 115
Medical Student's Disease 61
Meibomian 17
Memory lapses 31
Menstrual cycle 25
Methylcellulose 73
Michelson, Dr. Paul E. 75
Middle ear 25
Mikulicz' disease 56
Mixed connective tissue disease 36
Miyawaki, Dr. Shoji 105
Moisture Seekers, The 114, 115, 116, 117
Moisturizers 94
Mood swings 31
Morgan, Dr. Winfield, and Dr. Benjamin Castleman 59
Motter, Joyce 117
Mouth *see Dry mouth*
Moutsopoulos, Dr. H. M. 103, 106, 107, 110
Mucous glands 24, 25, 26, 28, 46
Mucus 29, 59
Mucus-dispersing (mucolytic) drops 76
Multiple sclerosis 52
Multipurpose Arthritis Center 104
Mumps 46
Muscles 8, 27, 30, 37, 38, 53, 88, 89
Muscular Dystrophy Association 122
Myositis 53, 95, 122
Napp 56

Nasal passages 24, 25, 35, 58
National Institute of Dental Research, NIH 105
National Institute of Arthritis and Metabolic Diseases 104
National Institute of Health (NIH) 105, 106, 108
National Lupus Erythematosus Foundation 122
National Organization for Rare Disorders (NORD) 121, 122
National Orphan Drug and Device Foundation 121
Natural History of Quackery, The 99
Natural killer (NK) cells 45
Nausea 29, 30
Neonatal lupus erythematosis (NLE) 35, 105, 112
Nerves 31, 37
New England Pathological Society 59
New York Chapter, SS Foundation 115
Nobel Prize for Medicine, 1950 84
Nocturnal lagothpthalmos. 18
Non-Steroidal Anti-Inflammatory Drug (NSAID) 8, 82
Northeast Ohio Chapter, SS Foundation 117

Index

Northern Imposter 99
Numbness 27
Nutrition 105
Ofuji, Dr. Tadashi 105
Ohio State University 127
Okayama University 105
Oldstone 107
Orphan Drug Act 122
Orphan drugs 121, 122
Ostler 104, 105
Ovaries 57
Pain 123
Pain receptors 89
Painful intercourse 26
Painkillers 68
Pancreas 27, 29, 30
Papas, Dr. Athena 116
Paracelsus, Dr. 99
Parotid flow rate 64
Parotid glands 22, 52, 59, 64, 67, 82
Pavlidis, Dr. N. 107
Penicillamine 86
Pennebaker, Jamie 127
People's Republic of China 106
Periotron 68
Peripheral Nervous Systems 31
Peripheral problems 95
Ph balance 50
Phagocytes 44, 45, 46
Phoenix Chapt., SSF 116
Phosphate 50
Phosphorus 20
Photosensitivity 18, 37, 77, 110
Pilocarpine 109
Pleurisy 24
Pneumonia 24
Polyarteritis 60
Polymers 93
Polymyositis 10, 13, 36, 38, 60
Polyvinyl alcohol 75
Post nasal drip 35
Prause, Dr. Jan Ulrik 62, 106, 107, 109, 110
Prednisone 8, 84, 85
Pregnancy 36
Preservatives 75
Primary Sjogren's syndrome 10, 13, 15, 16, 36, 37, 52, 53, 64, 82, 86
Prostaglandins 109
Protein 18, 34
Protozoa 44
Psuedo lymphomas 32
Punctal occlusion 76
Purpura 26, 53, 60
Quackery 99
RA factor 32, 70
Radiation 68
Random muscular jerks 31
Rashes 34, 112
Raynaud's phenomenon 27, 37, 45, 53
Recurring infections 25
Red blood cells 70
Redness 38
Refluxing 30, 96
Reichstein, Tadeus 84
Relaxation 93, 94, 126
Remineralise 20
Report on Fake Health Claims, Worthless Remedies, and Unproved Therapies, 101
Research 105-110
Restlessness 86
Retinal detachment 19

Rheumatoid arthritis (RA) 15, 23, 36, 52, 53, 69, 70, 71, 87, 108, 112, 125
Rhinitis 25
Ribbingska home in Lund, Sweden 58
Rose bengal staining 58
Rosen, Betty 5, 38
Royal College of Physicians and Surgeons of Glasgow 57
Ruhl, Helen 23, 112
Ruiz-Arguelles, Dr. Guillermo J. 20
Sagan, Dr. Carl 13
Saline tears 75
Saliva 5, 10, 20-22, 24, 29, 31, 46, 50, 51, 52, 53, 56, 57, 58, 60, 64, 65, 77, 79, 80, 81, 96, 109
Saliva substitutes 92
Schirmer test 58, 64, 65, 67, 69
Salivary glands 19, 22, 24, 32, 56, 57, 60, 64, 79-82, 105, 106
San Francisco's VA Hospital 104
Scandinavian Sjogren's group 106
Science Writers Seminar in Ophthalmology 110
Scintigram 63, 64
Sciubba, Dr. James 109, 115
Scleroderma 10, 12, 13, 36, 38, 60, 71, 89, 122
Scleroderma Assoc., Inc. 122
Scleroderma Federation 122

Scripps Clinic, 75, 107
Secondary Sjogren's syndrome 7, 10, 11, 15, 16, 23, 36, 37, 52, 53, 64, 70, 86, 120
Sed rate (erythrocyte sedimentation rate) test 70, 87
Self examination 33
Sensation of a foreign body in eyes 58
Sense of smell 25
Sense of touch 31
Serafimerlasarettet 57
Sex hormones 84, 108
Shearn, M. A. 11, 59, 107
Sheehy, Dr. Thomas, Jr. 25, 97
Shehi, Anita 115
Shimuzu, Dr. 119
Shortness of breath 24
Sialogram 64
Sicca City 13, 16, 22, 27, 32, 38
Sicca complex 52
Sight 56
Sjogren, Dr. Henrik 57, 58
Sjogren's Syndrome 11
Sjogren's Syndrome, A Dry-Eyed Diary 118
Sjogren's Syndrome, Clinical and immunological Aspects 103
Sjogren's Syndrome Clinic 104
Sjogren's Syndrome Foundation, Inc. 10, 104, 114-119, 122
Skin 24, 26, 27, 37, 38, 71, 84, 94, 95

Index

Slit lamp 65
Slow growing virus 44
Sluggishness 53
Sneezing 35
Sore throat 21
Southern Methodist University 127
Soviet Union 106
Speech difficulty 24
Spiera, Dr. Harry 116
Spleen 27
SS-A antibodies 51, 53, 69, 105
SS-B antibodies 57, 69
Stanford Arthritis Clinic 120
Steinberg, Dr. Alfred 108
Steroids 82, 84, 85, 86
Stiffness 23
Stomach 24, 28, 29, 30
Stress 24
Stuffiness 25, 34, 35
Sugai, Dr. Susumi 105, 118
Swallowing 20, 21, 30, 126
Sweden's University of Lund 107
Swedish Medical Association 58
Swedish Rheumatology Society 59
Swelling 22, 23, 28, 30, 31, 32, 34, 35, 37, 38, 52, 53
Synovial capsule 23, 87, 88
Synovitis 88
Systemic lupus erythematosis (SLE) 9, 10, 12, 13, 15, 36, 37, 48, 52, 53, 60, 69, 71, 88, 105, 108
T cells 45-50, 104

Talal, Dr. Norman 12, 32, 48, 103, 104, 105, 106, 108, 115, 119
Tarail, Jane 117
Tasting 22, 25
Tear glands 16, 17, 18, 19, 24, 31, 56, 57, 58, 73, 77
Tear pumps 77
Teeth 19, 20, 50, 68, 78, 80, 81
Testing 69
Thomas, Rose 117, 126
Thiocyanate 50
Throat 21, 22, 61, 76, 77, 126
Thursfield, Dr. 56
Thymus gland 47
Thyroid gland 27, 52, 53, 57
Tooth Decay 20
Toxins 46
Tranquilizers 68
Treatment 73-102
Tseng, Dr. Scheffer Chuei-Goong 110
Tucson Chapter, SSF 116
Tumors 32, 38, 56
Udell, Dr. Ira J. 116
Uhtoff, Dr. 56
Ulcers 21, 28, 29, 80, 85
United Scleroderma Foundation 122
University of California at San Francisco 104, 107
University of Copenhagen 62, 105
University of Gothenburg 58
University of Ioannina's Medical School 106

University of Ishikawa 105
University of Texas Health Science Center at Houston 9, 37, 110
University of Texas Health Science Center in San Antonio, Texas 49, 103
Vaginal area 24, 25, 26, 96, 97
Vaginitis 24, 96, 97
van Bijsterveld score 64
Van Mulders, Dr. Adolf 29
Vasculitis 18, 26, 53, 85
Virus 44, 45, 46
Vitamin A 77, 110
Vitamin D 84
Vitreous humor 18
Voice box 24
Von Grosz, Dr. 58
von Mikulicz-Radecki, Dr. Johann 56, 59, 60
Vulva 57
Waldenstrom's macroglobulinemia 112
Weakness 35, 37
Webs 30
Weight gain 84
Weight loss 34
Whitcher, Dr. John P. 105
White cells 31, *see lymphocytes, T Cells*
Wilmer Ophthalmological Institute 105
Witter, Dianne C. 93
Wrists 23, 31, 37
X-rays 70, 71
X-ray treatments 82
Xerophthalmia 63, 64
Xerosis 63
Xerostomia 19, 57, 64, 65, 91
Yeast infections 21

Having trouble explaining Sjogren's syndrome to your friends?
Want to bring your doctors up to snuff?
Want to spread the word and help the Sjogren's Syndrome Foundation at the same time?
(Part of this publication's profits is donated to the Foundation.)

Use order form below to send for more copies of

Sjogren's Syndrome
the Sneaky Arthritis

The ONLY book on Sjogren's syndrome written for patients by a fellow patient in easily understood language with a dollop of humor thrown in.

(Cut on this line)
YES! Please send me _____ copies of SJOGREN'S SYNDROME - The Sneaky "Arthritis" @ $11.95 ea., Postpaid. (Florida residents add $.60 sales tax).
Make check payable to Pixel Press.
Mail to: **Pixel Press**
            Dept. B
            P.O. Box 3151
            Tequesta FL 33469   Please print

Name_____

Street_____

City_____

State_____Zip_____
Sjogren's Syndrome Foundation Member?_____

Author's Note:

If **Sjogren's Syndrome,** the "Sneaky Arthritis" has been helpful or a comfort to you, please let me hear from you. Or if your experience with SS tops everything you've read here, I'd like to hear that, too! Maybe I can use your story in a future edition. Or I'd just like to keep in touch. Write me in care of the publisher at Pixel Press, PO Box 3151, Tequesta FL 33469.

                                        Sue Dauphin